Sarra Nasri
Sabra Jaâfoura

Optimizing the precision of ceramic veneers

Sarra Nasri
Sabra Jaâfoura

Optimizing the precision of ceramic veneers

The precision of ceramic veneers

ScienciaScripts

Imprint
Any brand names and product names mentioned in this book are subject to trademark, brand or patent protection and are trademarks or registered trademarks of their respective holders. The use of brand names, product names, common names, trade names, product descriptions etc. even without a particular marking in this work is in no way to be construed to mean that such names may be regarded as unrestricted in respect of trademark and brand protection legislation and could thus be used by anyone.

Cover image: www.ingimage.com

This book is a translation from the original published under ISBN 978-620-6-72088-1.

Publisher:
Sciencia Scripts
is a trademark of
Dodo Books Indian Ocean Ltd. and OmniScriptum S.R.L publishing group

120 High Road, East Finchley, London, N2 9ED, United Kingdom
Str. Armeneasca 28/1, office 1, Chisinau MD-2012, Republic of Moldova, Europe
Printed at: see last page
ISBN: 978-620-8-07251-3

Table of contents

Introduction

"Smile, because your teeth aren't just for eating or biting," proclaimed 20th-century filmmaker and photographer Man Ray (1).

Physical appearance, the cult of beauty and the quest for eternal youth are at the heart of today's society.

The aesthetics of the smile are an important part of this perpetual quest.

Dentists are increasingly called upon to provide aesthetic solutions to meet this growing demand.

Several treatment options are available to ensure the patient's aesthetic appeal.

Treating patients with ceramic veneers is a proven and reliable treatment option, offering a high success rate of around 93% over 15 years, while preserving as much of the healthy tooth structure as possible.

This therapy requires precision work both in the clinic and in the laboratory.

The word "precision" comes from the Latin "praecisio" and "-on", meaning the action of trimming.

According to Larousse, precision is defined as the character of what is precise.

The word "precise" comes from the Latin "praecisus", meaning "cut".

As well as suggesting the possibility of continuous improvement, this definition also evokes the idea of subjectivity.

According to Masseroni D et al (6) (Precision in Dental Esthetics): "It's not the elusive precision we're looking for, but rather the least degree of imprecision".

On the other hand, the concept of precision is closely linked to accuracy, a less reductive concept and therefore better suited to the complexity of prosthetic treatment. It may therefore be more productive to evaluate, in terms of precision, not only the dento-prosthetic joint, but also the operative steps, all conceived, planned and carried out at high magnification (6).

Since the 1970s(2) , dentists have been exploring the use of magnification in dentistry. At first, this use was dedicated to endodontics, then expanded to encompass all the other disciplines of dentistry

It can range from low magnification (2x-8x) to high magnification (16x-25x) (2).
It gives dentists a more detailed and precise view during treatment, contributing to more predictable results. As a result, the use of optical aids in dentistry is seen as a real revolution. The most ergonomic loupes were developed in the 1990s(3) , starting with an adjustable magnifier system and progressing to lighter loupes. The surgical microscope was introduced in the early 1920s (3).

The advent of digital technology has also transformed our practice. Digital technology provides solutions to a number of problems, ensuring smoother communication between the various parties involved (practitioner, prosthetist and patient).

With its cutting-edge technologies, digital technology enables us to control the smallest details of our work, giving dentists the opportunity to check themselves and make up for lost time on the spot.

In this work, we will attempt to review the microscopic and numerical tools available and their contribution to ceramic veneer processing (1,3 ,5).

1. Facets

1.1. Definition

Ceramic veneers are indirect, non-invasive aesthetic restorations for anterior teeth in need of aesthetic treatment.

They restore the vestibular surface of the tooth and part of the proximal and sometimes palatal surfaces (8,10).

1.2. Indications and contraindications for veneers

1.2.1. Indications (8,10)

- Tooth discoloration resistant to bleaching procedures.
- Morphological changes in the teeth (conoidal teeth).
- Diastema closure.
- Altered enamel structure (amelogenesis imperfecta, Huorosis, etc.).

1.2.2. Counter indications (9)

- Extensive carious lesions
- Poor oral hygiene.
- Teeth with insufficient enamel.
- The presence of parafunctions[8] .

1.3. Materials used for ceramic dental veneers

1.3.1. Ceramic classification

According to the American Society for Testing and Materials (9), a ceramic is a material, whether vitrified or not, with a crystalline or partially crystalline structure, or made of glass. Its body consists mainly of inorganic, non-metallic substances. It is formed either by solidification of a molten mass during cooling, or by a heat-induced forming and maturing process, simultaneously with or subsequent to its creation.

Practitioners are therefore faced with a multitude of possibilities. It is therefore necessary to have a classification that facilitates understanding and the choice of the most appropriate ceramic system. In 1995, Saadoun and Ferrari (9) proposed a classification of ceramics for metal-free prostheses.

This classification is based on two main criteria: the chemical composition of the ceramics and the shaping techniques used.

Indeed, the final characteristics of ceramics are the result of both the chemical composition of the material and the manufacturing process used, as illustrated in Table 1 (9).

Table 1: A classification of ceramics based on their composition and forming process, according to Saadoun and Ferrari (9).

Famille de céramique	Sous-famille composition		Usage		Mise en œuvre			Microstructure
			Armature	Monobloc	Pressée	Usinée	Barbotine	
Vitrocéramiques	Feldspath	Naturel ou synthétique	Non	Oui	Non	Oui (Vita Mark® II)	Non	
		Renforcé à la leucite	Oui	Oui	Oui (Empress® esthetic)	Oui (Empress® CAD)	Non	
	Disilicate de lithium		Oui	Oui	Oui (Emax® Press)	Oui (Emax® CAD)	Non	
Alumineuses infiltrées	Alumine-spinelle		Oui	Oui	Non	Oui (In-Ceram® Spinell)	Non	
	Alumine		Oui	Oui	Non	Oui (In-Ceram® Alumina)	Oui (In-Ceram® Alumina)	
	Alumine-zircone		Oui	Non	Non	Oui (In-Ceram® Zirconia)	Non	
Denses	Alumine dense		Oui	Non	Non	Oui (Procera® Alumine)	Non	
	Zircone Y-TZP		Oui	Oui « Full Zircone »	Non	Oui (Procera® Zircone, Lava®...)	Non	

Gracis in 2016[11] proposed a new classification following the introduction of so-called "hybrid" ceramics. (Figure 3).

According to this system, all-ceramic restorative materials can be grouped into three categories based on their chemical composition:

- Glass-matrix ceramics: these are non-metallic, inorganic ceramic materials containing a glassy phase.

- Polycrystalline ceramics: these are defined as inorganic, non-metallic ceramic materials that do not contain glass, but only a crystalline phase.
- Resin matrix ceramics: these are materials comprising a polymer matrix containing mainly inorganic refractory compounds[11] .

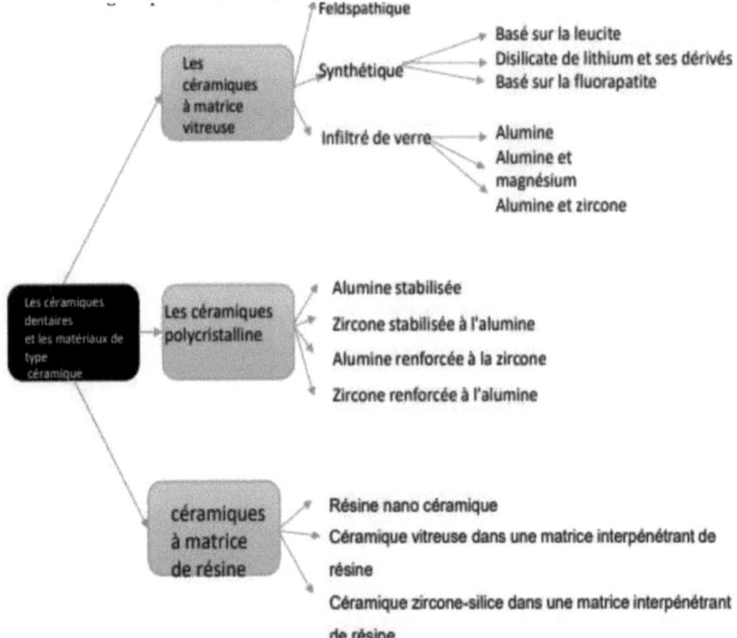

Figure 1: Ceramic classification by Gracis et al En 2016 [11]

1.3.2. Ceramics for dental veneers:

Although numerous ceramic systems are available, only some of them are suitable for dental veneers.

These ceramics must have good optical properties and a predominantly vitreous phase that can be etched to improve bondability.

The most commonly used ceramics are feldspathic ceramics, leucite-reinforced feldspathic ceramics and lithium disilicate ceramics (21). They can also be manufactured using alumina or zirconium oxide ceramics.

1.3.2.1. Feldspathic ceramics

Feldspathic ceramics are mainly composed of silica dioxide (60%-64%) and aluminum oxide (20%-23%).

Veneers are made using a layering technique that gives the technician total control, but requires a great deal of time and effort.

Advantages :

- Translucency close to natural tooth due to high glass content.
- Low laboratory costs compared with other ceramic systems.
- Excellent bonding characteristics after hydrofluoric acid etching and in the presence of an adequate amount of enamel.

Disadvantages :

- Poor mechanical properties (45).

1.3.2.2. Leucite-reinforced feldspathic ceramics (45)

Ceramics are composed of approximately 50% to 55% Ieucite crystals, homogeneously distributed in the glass matrix (Figure 4).

This material has a crystallinity level of 45% by volume, made up mainly of Ieucite fired at 1200° C, then pressed in molds and stabilized in its cubic form(45).

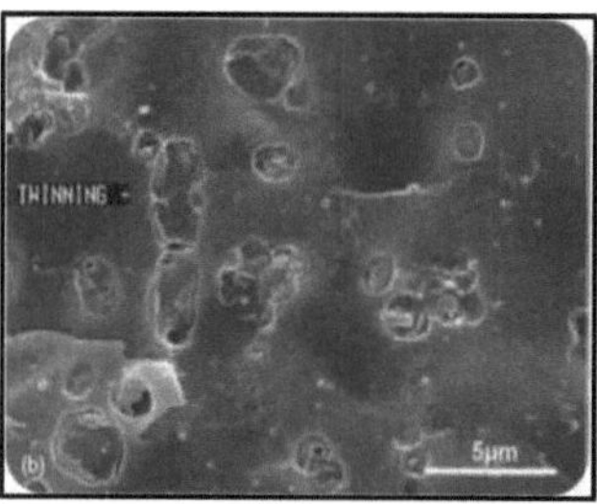

Figure 2:Scanning electron microscope view of a leucite-reinforced glass-ceramic (IPS Empress) [12]

1.3.2.3. Lithium disilicate-reinforced ceramics

Ceramics contain 70% lithium discilicate crystals (IPS Empress II and currently

IPS Emax).

Lithium disilicate-based ceramics offer better resistance to fracture, thermal shock and corrosion.

The platelet-like microstructure of lithium disilicate crystals requires shaping in a partially crystallized state, with a lithium metasilicate proportion of 40% by volume. In this state, the material has a flexural strength of 130 MPa and the blocks can be easily machined. The final microstructure of the material is controlled by heat treatment (sintering) (Figure 5) (45).

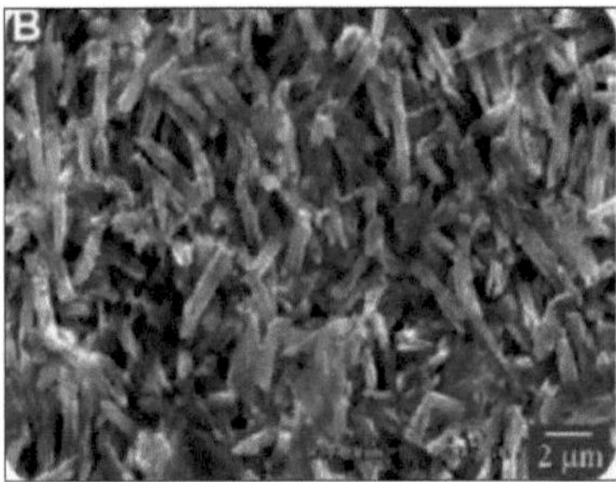

Figure 3: Scanning electron microscope view of a lithium disilicate ceramic (IPS E max) [12]

1.3.2.1. Alumina-based ceramics[10] :

Alumina-based ceramics are sintered ceramics.

Depending on its composition, In-ceram ceramic is classified as In-ceram alumina, In-ceram spinel and In-ceram zirconia.

1.3.2.1.1. In-ceram alumina

It is composed of 85% aluminum oxide particles. This high alumina content confers a flexural strength of 400 to 600 MPa.

In-ceram alumina ceramics offer higher strength and fracture toughness than feldspathic ceramics.

1.3.2.1.2. Spinelle In-ceram

In-ceram spinel contains a mixture of magnesia and alumina (MgA1204) in its structure to increase its translucency. Its flexural strength is lower than that of In-ceram alumina.

1.3.2.1.3. In-ceram zirconia

This is a modification of the original In-ceram alumina, composed of 67% aluminum oxide and 33% zirconium oxide.

It has a fracture toughness and tensile strength of 600 to 800 MPa.

Its opaque character indicates a layer of cosmetic feldspathic ceramic.

1.3.2.2. Zirconia-based ceramics

The main characteristic of polycrystalline zirconia-based ceramics is a fine-grained crystalline structure offering resistance and fracture toughness, but tending to have limited translucency. In addition, the absence of a glassy phase makes polycrystalline ceramics difficult to etch with hydrocortic acid, requiring longer etching times or higher temperatures.[10][11]

1.3.3. Choice of materials for veneer fabrication

For ceramic veneers, the two most common material choices are lithium disilicate-reinforced ceramics (IPS e.max®) and feldspathic ceramics. In some cases, veneers made of composite resin or hybrid materials may also be indicated.

Lithium disilicate ceramics offer several advantages over feldspathic ceramics:

- flexural strength ranging from 360 to 400 MPa (compared with 90 to 100 MPa for feldspathic ceramics),
- a minimum thickness of only 0.3 mm (instead of 0.5 mm for feldspathic ceramics)
- better masking of discoloured teeth.

Despite the many advantages of lithium disilicate ceramics, feldspathic ceramics are often the appropriate choice when a single veneer is indicated to match strongly characterized natural teeth or an existing feldspathic ceramic restoration.

It is important to bear in mind that when choosing a suitable material, the practitioner must also consider the skills and limitations of the prosthetist, as each material may behave differently in different hands[10] .

Table 2: Comparison of the properties of ceramics used in dental veneers[10] ,

Materials	translucency	Flexural strength	Trade name
Feldspathic	Very important	60to70MPa	
Leucite-reinforced feldspar	Depending on the chemical composition and quantity of crystals incorporated in the matrix.	160 to 300 MPa	empress I
Lithium disilicate		320to450 MPa	empress II IPS emax Press IPS emax CAD
In-ceram alumina	Low translucency	400to 600MPa	alumina In-ceram
Spinelle In-ceram	Low translucency	<400MPa	
In-ceram zirconia	Lack of translucency	600to 800 MPa	In-ceram zirconia
Zirconia-based ceramics	Opaque		

2. Diagnosis and clinical data collection: the conventional chain

2.1. Aesthetic analysis:

2.1.1. The prosthetic project[1314] :

The wax-up is the three-dimensional materialization of a morphological proposal for the prosthesis by modeling in wax or using digital tools on the model and/or file from the arch impression.

It enables :

- Transfer esthetic designs and create the silicone key -Display the contours of target esthetic restorations using the mock-up. -Create temporary restorations.

2.1.2 The Mock up:

This is a resin model made preoperatively from the silicone key. It is used to check the aesthetics and function of the intraoral restoration[14] .

3. The treatment plan

3.1. Preparation for ceramic veneers

Preparations for ceramic veneers must ensure optimal marginal fit of the restoration while preserving hard dental tissue as far as possible.

Preparation must be limited to the enamel in terms of periphery and depth.

In some cases, the preparation may reach the incisal edge or the interproximal spaces.

Controlling the amount of reduction during the dental veneer preparation stage is a major concern for practitioners. Guided dental reduction has provided a solution to ensure uniform space for dental restoration without affecting pulpal and periodontal health, aesthetics and structural integrity. [8 14]

3.1.1. Contribution of calibrated strawberries :

To guarantee precise control of the preparation depth, special burs are available which allow calibration to the material used, depending on the clinical situation. Taking into account the average enamel thickness values of the Vestibular anterior teeth, these calibrated burs ensure sufficient preparation without risk of dentine exposure. A recommended sequence of instruments for controlled preparation of ceramic veneers (Figure 6)[22] :

- Countersink with depth stop.
- Long-necked ball diamond cutter.
- Double-granulated diamond milling cutter.
- Diamond milling cutter with rounded tip

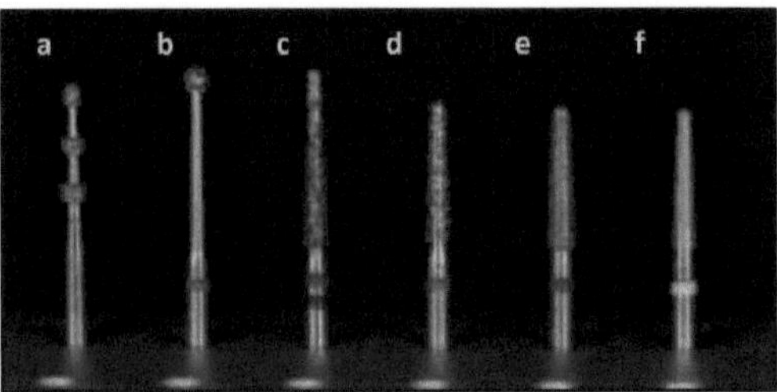

Figure 4:The burs recommended for preparing ceramic veneers for bonding: a: countersink b : long-necked ball diamond burr c :double-granulation diamond burr d , e ,f :¼-round conical diamond burr [22]

All milling cutter specifications are available in Table 3.

Table 3: Characteristics of facet preparation burs [22]

Objective	Name	Color code	Cutter diameter [ISO]	Penetration depth
Controlled preparation	Countersink with countersink stop		2.00mm	0.4mm
	Long neck ball end mill	Green	1.8mm	0.4mm
Preparation	Diamond milling cutter with rounded tip	Green	1.15mm at end	0.55mm
	Double granulation diamond milling cutter	Green/red	1.15mm end	0.55mm
	Diamond milling cutter with rounded tip	Red	1.15mm end	0.55mm
	Diamond milling cutter with rounded tip	Yellow	1.15mm end	0.55mm

For guided preparation, start by marking the depth using a long-necked ball end mill or a countersink. (Figure 7).

At this stage, the parallelism between the mandrel and the surface must be respected. When preparing the incisors, it is essential to take into account the two axes Vl and V2, while a third axis, V3, is also present at canine level. Compliance with these axes ensures optimum preparation of the vestibular surface. (Figure 8).

Thanks to the conical shape of its active part and its rounded tip, the countersink has the advantage of preventing excessive penetration, even when the instrument is tilted excessively (Figure 9).

At the free edge, vertical grooves are made using a diamond burr with a rounded tip over its entire cross-section to guarantee the necessary space of over 1.5 mm for the ceramic in this area. (Figure 10).

-The resulting grooves are marked out with a graphite pencil and then joined together using a fillet-type cutter with a rounded tip, taking care not to penetrate beyond half their thickness (Figure 11).

The use of a special burr with double granulation avoids any over-separation at cervical level. One end has a fine red-ring granulometry, the rest a normal green-ring granulometry.

- Gingival extensions are created beyond the gingival papillae using the toboggan principle. This makes it possible to mask the veneer limits on a profile view. (Figure 12).

The cervical margin should always be supra-gingival, or even juxta-gingival in the presence of pronounced dental dyschromia, in order to facilitate placement of the surgical field and, consequently, bonding. (Figure 3)[2214] .

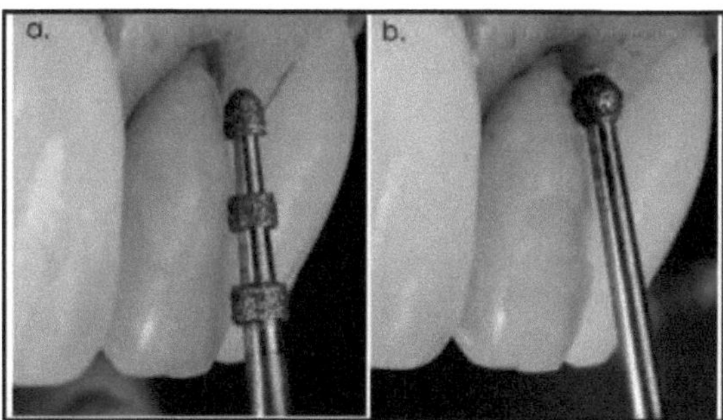

Figure 5: a: Countersink with countersink stop b: Long neck ball end mill [22]

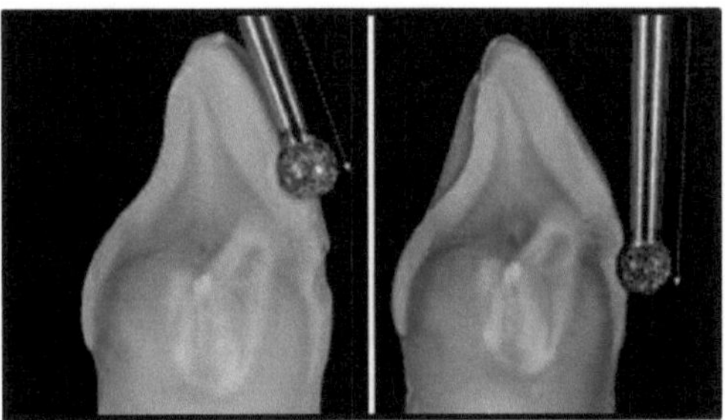

Figure 6: The two tooth axes V1 and V2 [22]

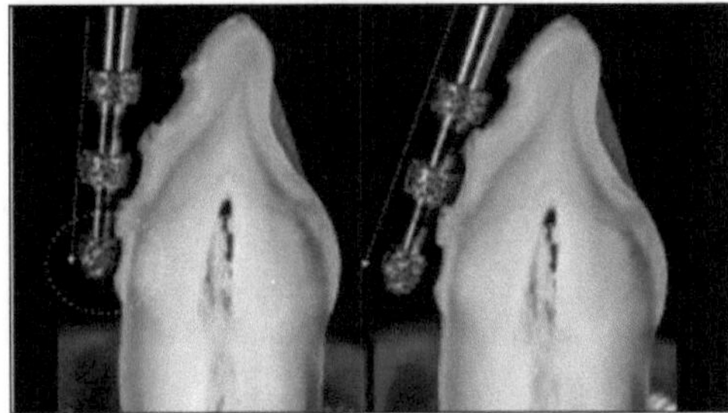

Figure 7: Preparing the vestibular surface with the countersink along axes V1 and V2 [22]

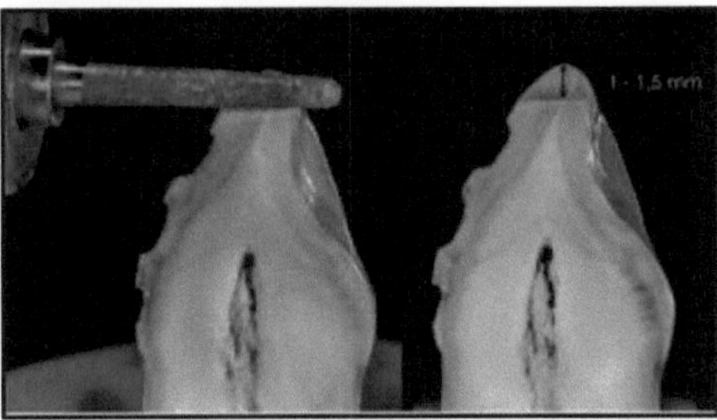

Figure 8: Preparing the free edge [22]

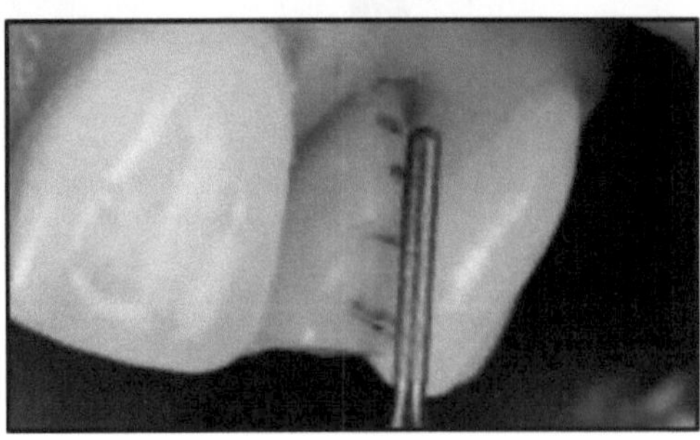

Figure 9:The round-ended fillet cutter connects the grooves until the pencil lines disappear. [22]

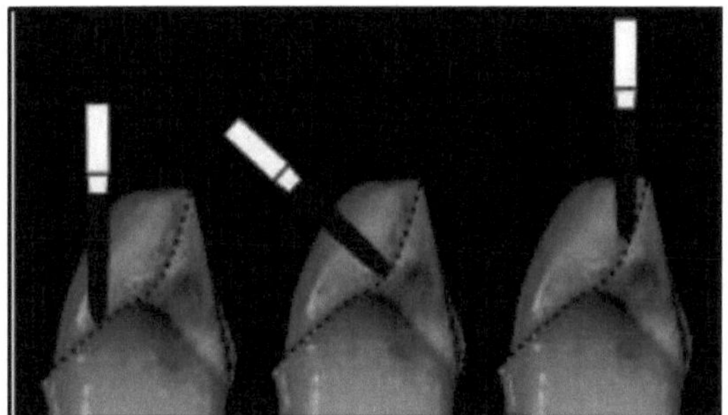

Figure 10: Gingival-proximal extensions beyond the papillae [22]

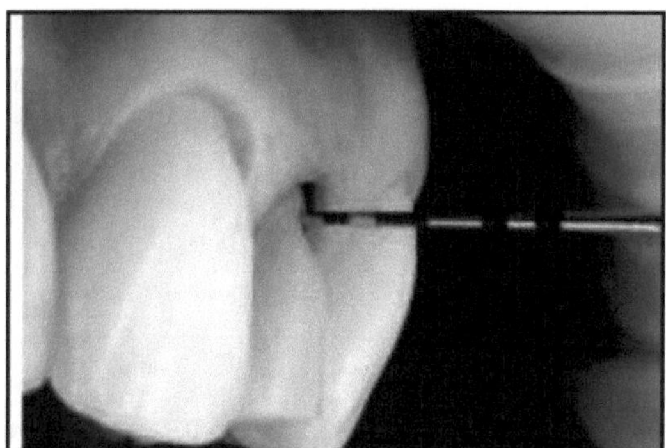

Figure 11: Profile view of supragingival preparation margin [22]

3.1.2. Preparation through mock-up

The mock-up is an acrylic resin mask transferred into the mouth using a silicone key made on the wax-up-corrected model. The tooth preparation guide is an auxiliary tool used in the tooth preparation process. Its main purpose is to quantify and visualize the space between the preparation and the tooth surface[14].

In other words, it allows you to visualize the aesthetic project in your mouth. After any necessary balancing and aesthetic and functional validation, this guide can be used to ensure that the preparation is as conservative as possible.

The silicone key is cut and adjusted to follow the contour of the scalloped gum line (Figure 14).

It is then filled with resin and applied to the teeth with pressure in the Occlusal direction while any excess resin is removed (Figure 15).[23] .

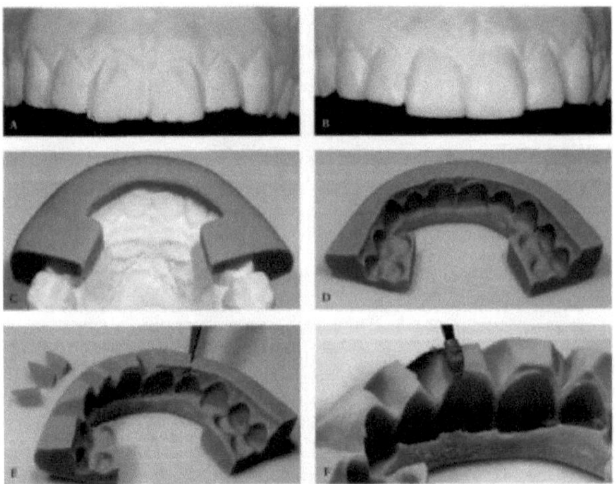

Figure 12: Preparing the silicone key [23]

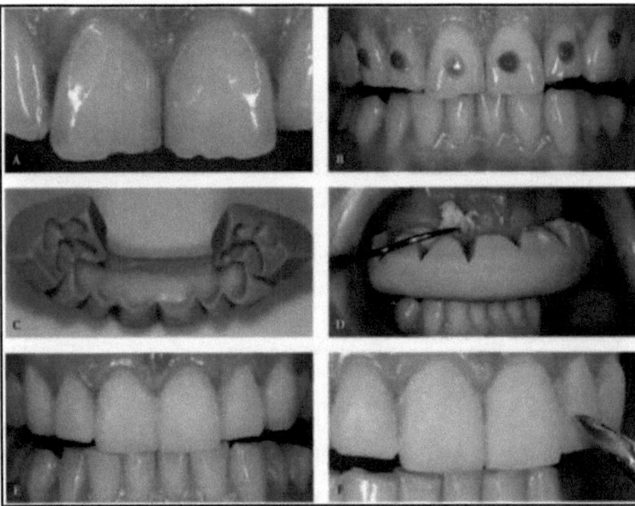

Figure 13: Preparing the reduction key (32) :

To prepare the teeth, we start by creating two grooves: a horizontal one at mid-height on the outer surface of the tooth, and a scalloped one between the middle and cervical thirds. We then use a round-ended diamond bur to progressively remove the remaining tooth substance between these grooves.

We check the available reduction space using the silicone key.

All corners are then rounded using the ultra-fine diamond disk (Figure 6).[23] .

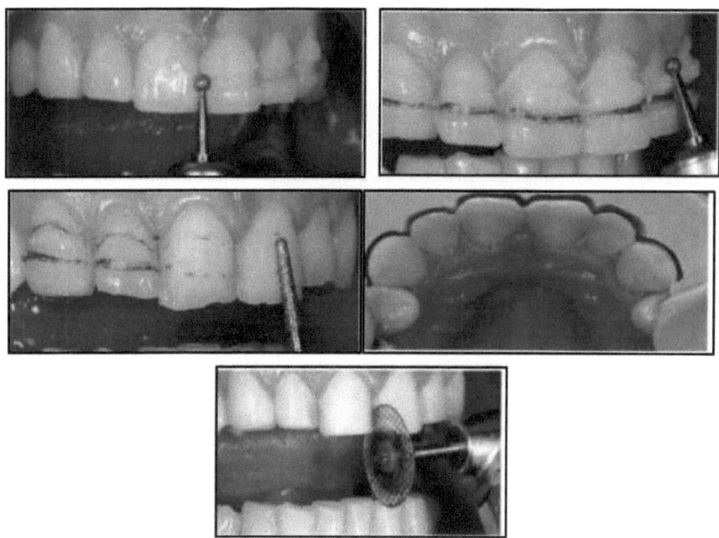

Figure 14: Tooth preparation[23] :

3.1.3. Reduction control keys

Various types of silicone reduction wrench can be used as a reduction guide. The two most common types are the window wrench and the vertical wrench[22] .

-The window wrench is generally used to determine the depth of preparation of anterior teeth for veneer restorations (Figure 17).

This key is made by removing the silicone from one cúspide to the other, at approximately
3 mm from the incisal edges. This "window" makes it possible to visualize the depth of facial and lingual preparation at approximately the level of the incisal and middle thirds of the tooth.
It is easy to make for upper and lower front teeth[22] .

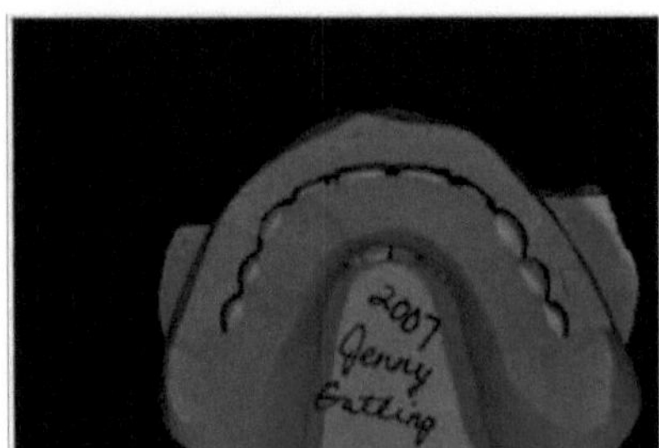

Figure 15: The window wrench [22]

-The vertical wrench is a highly versatile index. It can be used effectively in all areas of the mouth. It is simple in design and extremely effective in controlling reduction depth.

A vertical index is created by simply cutting the horseshoe-shaped silicone index vertically through the center of the tooth to be evaluated (Figure 18). Ensuring that the index is correctly supported by the adjacent teeth, tooth preparation can be assessed by visualizing the restorative space created in relation to the wax contours captured by the index. Over- or under-reduction can be easily assessed. Multiple vertical cuts are possible with a single index[22] .

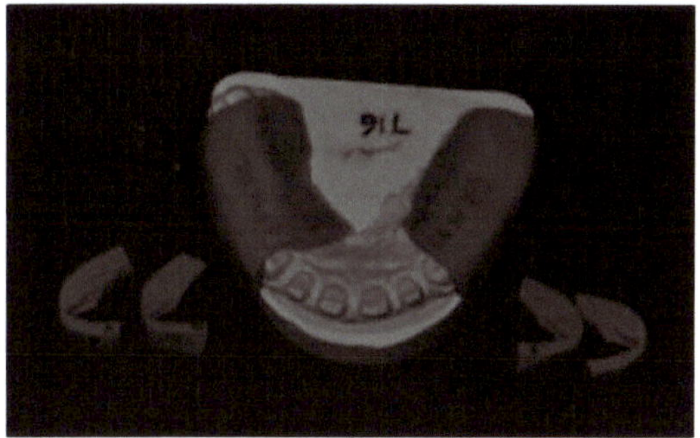

Figure 16: The vertical reduction key [22]

3.1. The choice of color

Precise color selection is crucial.

Harmonizing the color of ceramic veneers with the remaining teeth is of paramount importance to patients. Color can be determined by visual assessment or by measuring the three dimensions of color according to Mursell: hue, saturation and brightness.

-Hue is the quality that differentiates one family of colors from another, for example, red from yellow.

-Luminosity is used to distinguish a light color from a dark one. It's a value measured on a scale ranging from black to white, with gradations of gray. Saturation is the intensity of hue[15Д6].

3.1.1. What you need to know before choosing a color

The color that appears depends on the light source or lighting.

Use color-corrected lighting and avoid bright colors in the work area.

The practitioner should avoid bright colors in the work area.

- Natural light between 10 a.m. and 2 p.m. is the best light source for color harmonization, but it is unreliable due to its variable color temperature, which affects its spectral composition. It may be useful to use an auxiliary light source that provides the appropriate spectral balance and diffuse illumination, and is bright enough to overcome the effects of ambient lighting.

If the patient is wearing light-colored clothing, cover with a gray sheet.

- Dark lipstick should be removed prior to shade selection. Similarly, the tooth-colour selection procedure should always start with clean teeth.

-If lightening is envisaged, it should be carried out at least 2 weeks before color selection to minimize regression effects.

- The shade tab must lie in the same plane as the tooth, either above or below the tooth to be matched.
- A second observer stands about 3 feet behind the main observer to check that the color is appropriate.
- Photographs taken with well-defined equipment are essential: nothing else can provide valuable information like the degree of translucency, the size and shape of incisal nipples, and other individual characteristics of teeth[171816].

3.1.2. Conventional shades of color choice [15]

Always check with your dental technician regarding the type of ceramic used and the shade guide chosen.

3.1.2.1. Vitapan classique (Vita Zahnfabik)

Vitapan Classique was introduced with 16 tabs which are divided into four groups according to hue known as the A-to-D arrangement, and within each group there are four tabs which are divided according to saturation. (Figure 19).

Even though this guide is made of acrylic resin, it has been the reference guide in dentistry for decades '[1819].

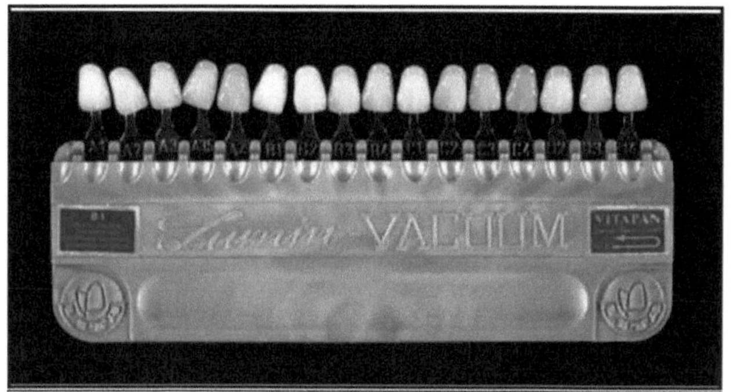

Figure 17: Vitapan classic shade guide [18]

3.1.2.1. Vitapan 3D master shade system (Vita)

The shade guide is organized to cover the three-dimensional color of the natural tooth in a logical, visually equidistant sequence. It provides virtually all existing natural tooth shades. It has been determined that the order of color dimensions in this guide is appropriate.

The tabs are divided into five clearly perceptible brightness levels. Within each level, tabs represent different saturations and hues.

The brightest brightness level (group 1) has only two saturation levels of a single hue, and the darkest brightness level (group 5) has three saturation levels of a single hue.

Groups 2, 3 and 4 have three saturation levels in the middle hue (the orange hue) and two saturation levels in each hue moving towards yellow or red (Figure 20).

The color matching process is divided into three steps:

-The first is to select the nearest luminosity.

-In the second step, the saturation level is determined. This is generally easy, as each brightness group has its own saturation levels within the group.

-The third and final step is to determine the shade.

Consequently, each color is determined by a number (brightness), a letter (hue) and a number (saturation), as in the example 4M3, where 4 represents brightness,

M represents hue and 3 represents chroma '[1618] .

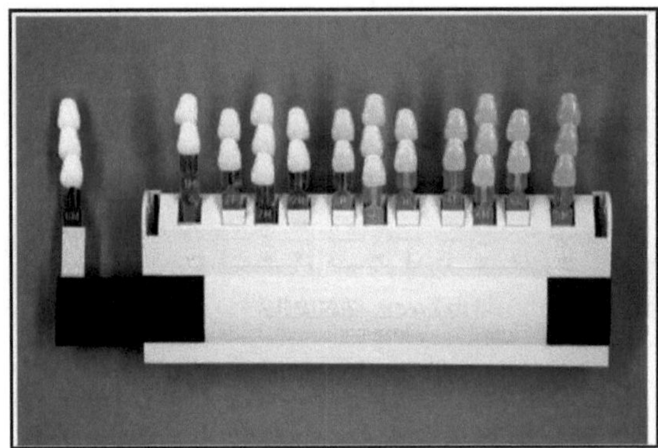

Figure 18: Vitapan 3D-Master shade guide [18]

3.1.2.1. Linear guide 3D master

This is a modification of vitapan 3D master. It contains exactly the same tabs, but with a simplified layout and a two-step shading procedure.

The shade guide holders contain only 6 to 7 linearly arranged tabs, comprising one brightness guide and five saturation/hue guides, each with three to seven tabs.

According to the manufacturer's instructions, the tooth matching procedure is divided into two steps. Firstly, the brightness group is selected using the brightness guide containing 3D tabs with medium saturation and neutral hue. Each brightness tab has a corresponding saturation/hue guide. In the second step, the user then determines the correct saturation and hue (figure 21)[19] .

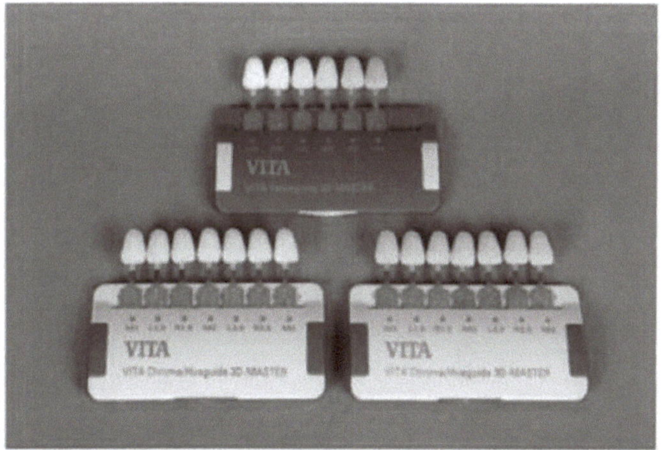

Figure 19: Linearguide 3D-Master[20] : the brightness guide is shown in the top row, and two of the five hue guides with the respective brightness in the bottom row.

3.2. Conventional footprint

3.2.1. Definition

The impression is a negative recording of all or part of the dental arch and its surrounding tissues. The aim is to ensure the most accurate possible transfer of all the anatomical elements recorded in the mouth to the laboratory for the production of positive models, which are faithful replicas of the tissues recorded (Figures 22 and 23)([24]).

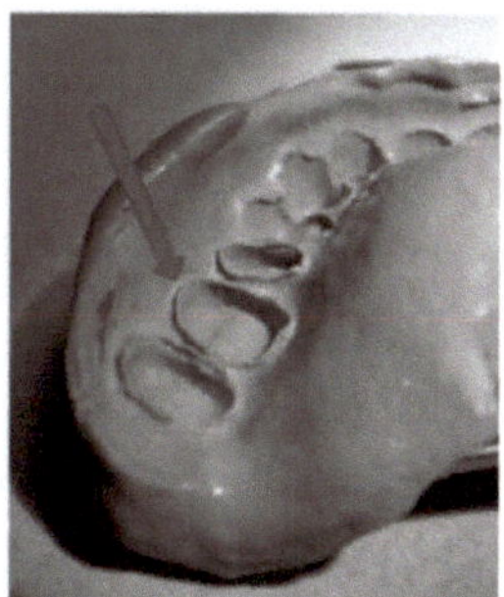

Figure 20: Simultaneous double-mix cavity[25]

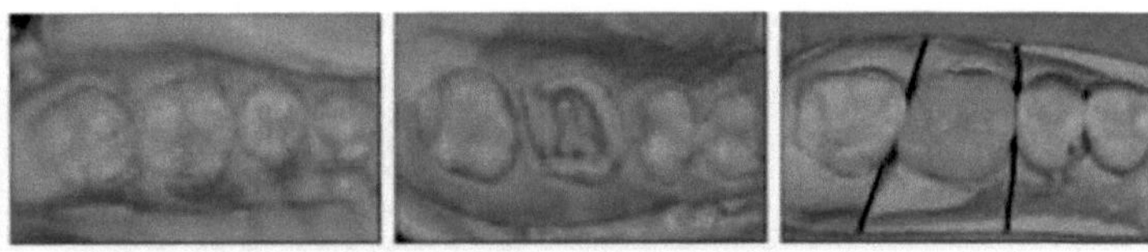

Figure 21: Conventional impression for stratified E maxPress Onlay[26]

3.2.2. Conditions for successful imprinting

-Hard tissue (prepared teeth, unprepared teeth) and soft tissue (periodontium) must be recorded as faithfully as possible. The impression must be made in a saliva-free environment.

-Perfect visibility of the finishing line.

-Absence of blood, saliva or fluid Sulcular[26]

3.2.3. The qualities required for an ideal impression material are :

- Easy handling
- Long working time, but short setting time in the mouth
- Hydrophilic and moisture tolerant
- Precise reproduction of details
- Immediate and delayed dimensional stability
- Tear strength
- Disinfection possible
- Compatibility with reproduction materials
- Reasonable cost

-Precision: elastomeric impression materials used to manufacture precision moldings must be able to reproduce fine details of 25 µm or less.

-Wettability of the impression material. Impression materials must be able to flow easily into details of 20 to 70 µm, which is necessary to obtain perfectly fitting impressions.

-Flexibility: flexible impressions are easier to remove from the mouth It's important to have an impression material that's flexible enough to overcome the undercuts of adjacent teeth and other intraoral structures.

25 27

3.3. Facet bonding

Once the ceramic veneers are ready, they are fitted and bonded.

- A dental dam is required to keep the field dry and clean during bonding procedures.
- Temporary restorations and all traces of temporary cement are removed to allow precise placement (Figure 24).

- Teeth are thoroughly cleaned with chlorhexidine gluconate disinfectant solution.
- Each veneer is carefully tried in and checked for fit, contacts and esthetics, as well as any excess or deficiencies that may occur at margin level. Proximal contacts and incisal edges must also be checked and adjusted to ensure that the veneers fit properly.
- A "Try In" gel is used to check the choice of bonding resin.

- The inside of the veneers should be rinsed and cleaned after fitting to remove any remaining material.

Once all these steps have been completed for each facet, the actual gluing begins.

Treatment of the intrados of veneers :

- The intrados of the veneers are etched with 2% hydrofluoric acid for 15 seconds, then rinsed for 20 seconds and dried.

- After a good rinse, they are silanized. The silane is left in contact with the intrados for 1 minute, then dried with an air syringe.
- Using a brush, the adhesive (Optibond 2FL adhesive; Kerr Corp., Orange, CA) is applied to the inside of the veneers. It is spread with the air spray before polymerization.

Treatment of dental surfaces:

- Teeth must be thoroughly cleaned after the trial phase.
- The tooth surface is then etched with 35% orthophosphoric acid for 15 seconds (Figure 25).
- They are then rinsed for 20 seconds and gently dried (Figure 26).
- Adhesive is applied to the prepared surfaces (Figure 27).
- An air jet is applied to ensure uniform coating.
- Photopolymerization for 20s.

We begin to set up the facets:

The veneers are placed on a veneer organizer in the order of the natural dentition and bonding begins one by one.

- Bonding resin is applied and each restoration is cured for 30 seconds per surface (Figure 28).
- The excess around the restorations is removed under magnification (Figure 29).
- Once all materials have been removed, teeth and tissues are cleaned with moist gauze[28] .

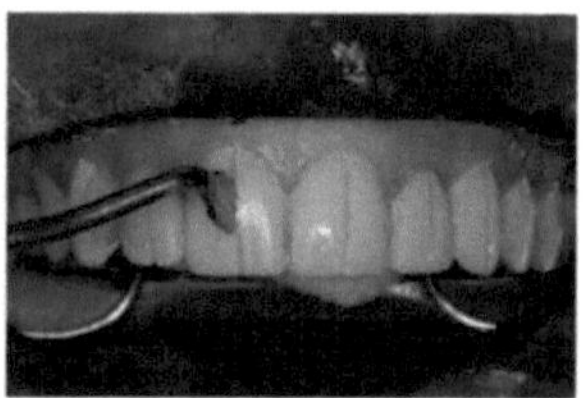

Figure 22: Removing temporary restorations( )[28]

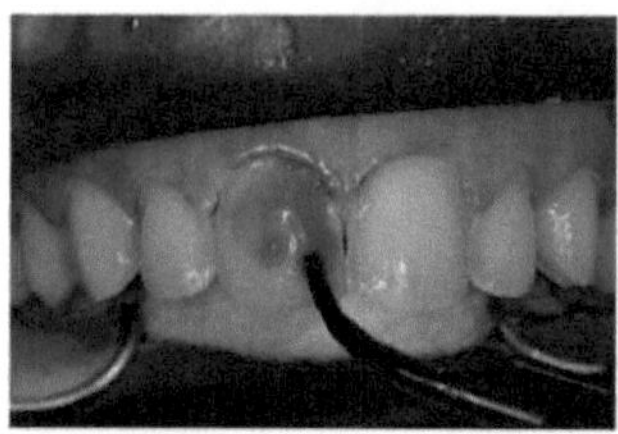

Figure 23: Applying orthophosphoric acid to the tooth surface( )[28]

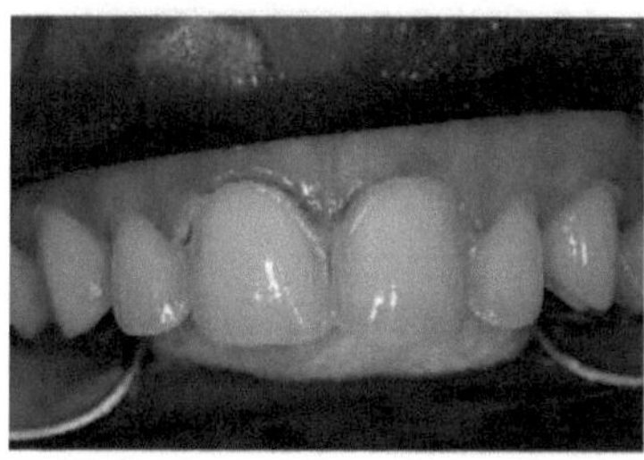

Figure 24: Rinsing and drying the teeth for 20s( )[28]

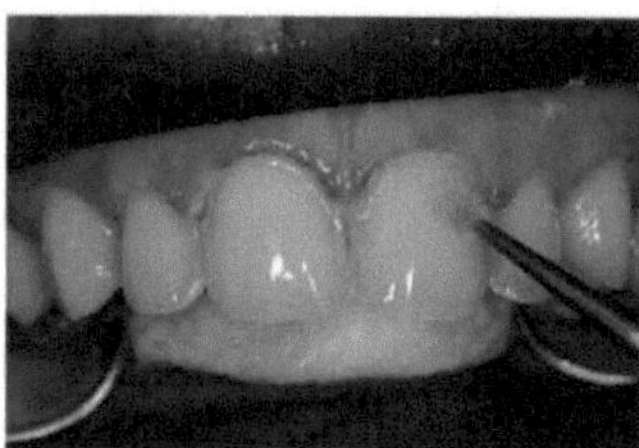

Figure 25: Applying adhesive to tooth surface( )[28]

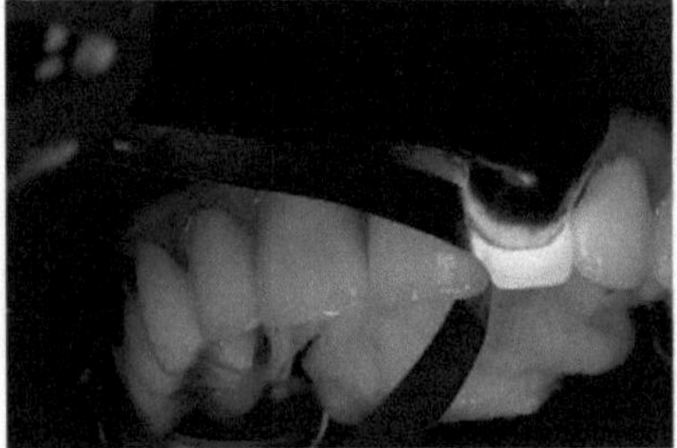

Figure 26: Light-curing( )[28]

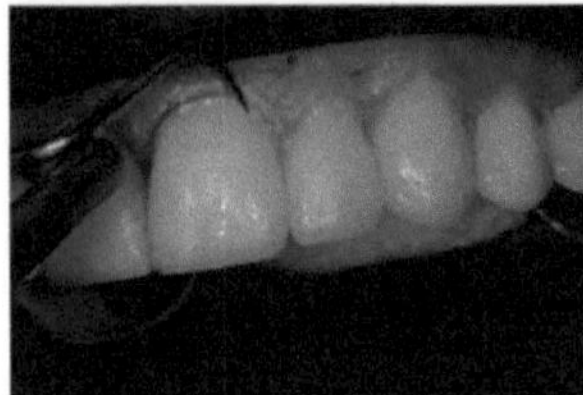

Figure 27: Removing excess material with absorbent cotton( )[28]

3.4. Effect of bonding on final veneer color

The color of a ceramic veneer is determined by several factors, including the color and thickness of the veneer, the thickness and color of the adhesive and finally the underlying tooth substrate.

Each resin is supplied with a trial paste to give a visual indication of the color of the final restoration before final bonding.

Some bonding sets are supplied with a trial paste to help the practitioner assess the color of the final veneers.

In order to provide a guide to the resin shade needed to achieve an acceptable restoration, the try-in paste must give an accurate reflection of the final color that will be achieved by this resin shade.

The veneers were applied to the teeth using trial pastes and the color was measured. They were then loaded with resin cement and placed on the prepared tooth surface.

It has been shown that a significant change in color can occur during the polymerization of the bonding resin, and the practitioner must take this into account when selecting the shade. However, there was a relative change in color between uncured and cured resin cements for all shades and all manufacturers.

These small color differences occurring during resin cement polymerization could be due to the reduced absorption of blue light by photoinitiators after light-curing. Color changes in resin cements during polymerization are not clinically significant, so unpolymerized resin cement can be used as a test paste.

In conclusion, the color adjustment obtained with the test paste should be treated with caution, and further evaluation of the restoration made with the resin in place before curing is recommended.[29]

I- Digital tools for optimizing the precision of ceramic veneers

1. Digital aesthetic design for ceramic veneers

For several years now, the advent of computer-aided design and manufacturing (CAD/CAM) and the dematerialization of certain stages in the prosthetic chain have revolutionized our professional practice.

The digital workflow ensures codification of the transfer of the various files, resulting in time and precision savings. This applies especially to ceramic veneers, where precision is of the utmost importance.

- In the study phase, the optical scanners digitize the initial condition of the oral cavity (maxillary arch, mandibular arch and occlusion records) into a digital file in standard tessellation language (STL) format. (Fig. 30.A).
- STL diagnostic data and the patient's extra-oral frontal photograph are imported into computer-aided design software, overlaying the photograph with the digitized maxilla. (Figure 30.B).

For accurate orientation of the casts, care must be taken to ensure that the patient's head is in the natural position when the photos are taken.

- At this stage, a digital wax-up is performed on the surfaces of the maxillary anterior teeth, according to the patient's aesthetic and functional parameters. (Figure 31.A and 32). This wax-up is identical to a conventional wax-up on a plaster model. It creates a 3D representation of the proposed result on the study model.
- A trial restorative guide is fabricated from bisacrylic resin and condensation silicone to evaluate esthetic and functional parameters (Figure 31.B) ([30]).

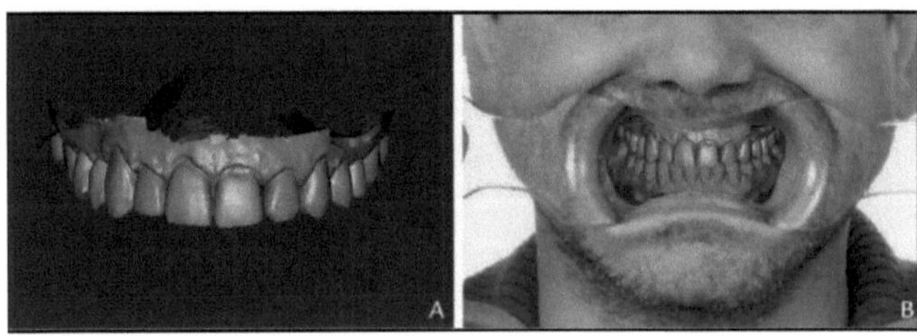

Figure 28: A :An STL file of the maxilla B :A photograph of the arches in occlusion superimposed on an initial STL file [30]

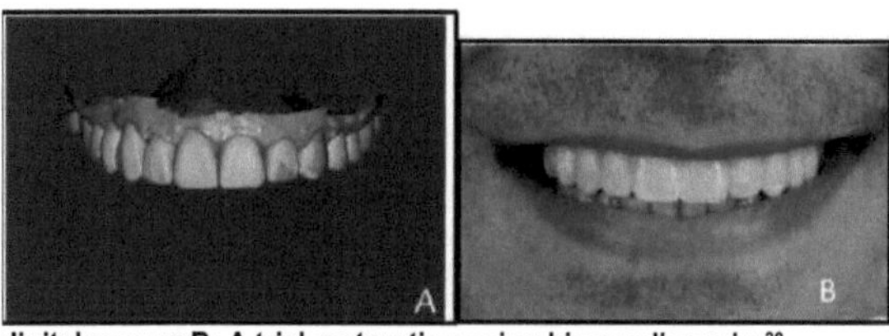

Figure 29: A: A digital wax-up B: A trial restoration using bis acrylic resin [30]

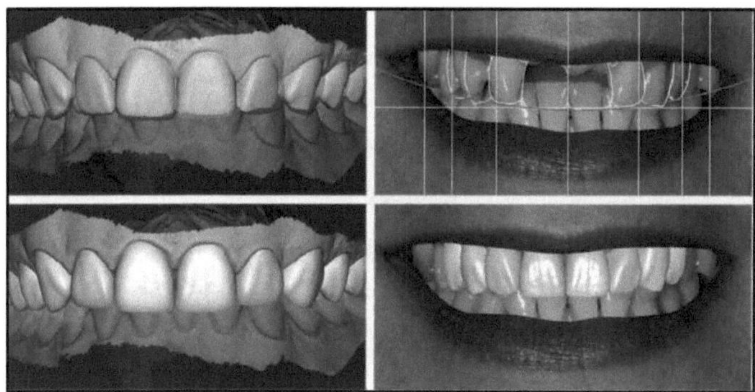

Figure 30: Digital smile design for mock-ups [31]

2. 3D-printed, CAD/CAM-designed preparation guides:

The use of 3D-printed reduction guides is an innovative technique that ensures improvements in precision when preparing dental veneers.

It's a resin guide additively manufactured to selectively reduce tooth surfaces.
The mock-up is used to evaluate aesthetic and functional parameters in the mouth. Once the mock-up has been validated intraorally, the digital preparation guide is designed. It enables more controlled, selective and non-invasive preparation, based on the approved trial restoration and limited to the minimum thickness required for definitive ceramic restorations.
After the necessary intra-oral adjustments, a new scan of the maxilla is taken and

the corresponding STL file is used to create the reduction guide.

A wax-up STL file and an initial STL file are imported and superimposed in design software.

Taking into account the minimum thickness required for the veneers, a virtual preparation is created, reducing the final volume compared to the STL wax-up file. We design a 2.0 mm thick structure covering the entire dental arch, with an offset distance of 0.05 mm, and create an open access to the dental surfaces in the initial STL file, which extrudes the wax-up STL file and then creates sleeved windows on the extruded surfaces.

Access windows for rotary instruments improve the accuracy of the amount of structure and limit the movement of the rotary instrument.

The literature shows that these 3D printed ones can be successfully used to evaluate specific surfaces such as incisal edges, axial and proximal faces however, no guide has been designed to evaluate multiple surfaces at the same time[30 ,32] .

1.1. Control guides for the vestibular surface :

The 3D printing guide plate transforms esthetic analysis and designed digital results into physical entities using 3D printing technology. It plays an important role in providing early insight into the aesthetic restoration and its precise implementation. This approach reduces steps such as model preparation and manual production of the aesthetic diagnostic wax model. This effectively improves the diagnostic rate and patient comfort.

Vestibular face reduction guides are divided into two types: equal-thickness guide plates and non-equal-thickness guide plates.

Equal thickness guide plates manufactured by 3D printing are equal in thickness. However, when using the depth control hole, the depth required to maintain different reduction zones must be different.ffigure 33).[14]

To simplify the depth control steps, 3D printed guide plates can be manufactured as non-equal thickness plates. In this way, the depth of the depth-calibrated milling cutter in the guide plate remains consistent in each preparation zone, and the depth-control preparation process is simplified (figure 34).[14]

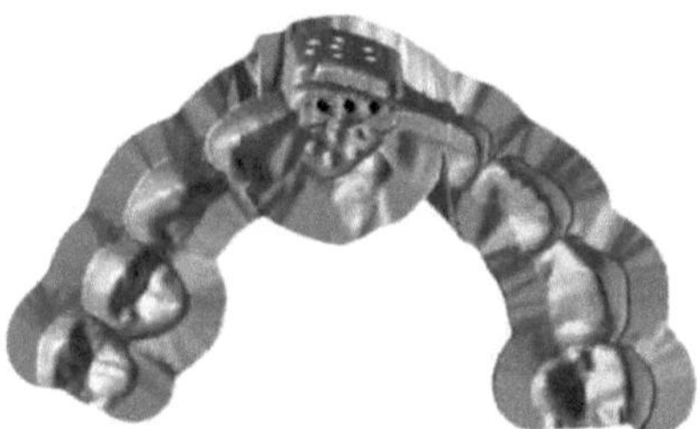

Figure 31: Three-dimensional impression of a guide plate for targeted restorative space of equal thickness [14]

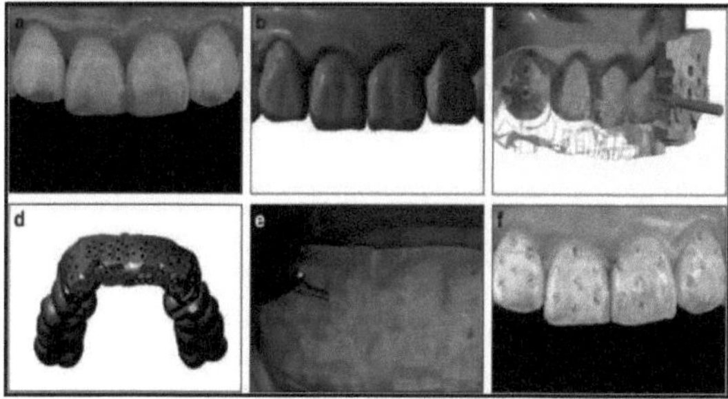

Figure 32: Three-dimensional (3D) printing of a guide plate with a targeted restorative space of unequal thickness for tooth preparation[14].

In some cases, the guides play a dual role as reduction guides for preparation and gingivectomy guides. They are used to ensure accurate gingivectomy and to assess the amount of reduction required. (figure 35)[33].

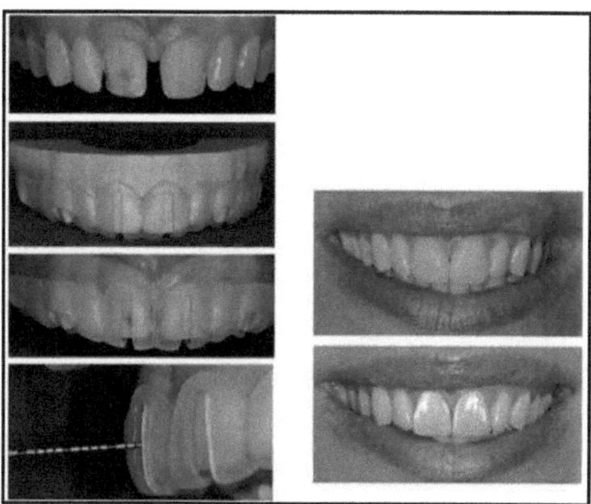

Figure 33: A 3D-printed dental reduction guide [33]

1.2. Incisal reduction control guides :

1.3. Multi-sided reduction guides

both :

With the advance of digital dentistry and versatile design software, guides can be created for all reduction planes, i.e. labial, vestibular and incisal, enabling conservative and, above all, good quantity preparations. These guides are printed in 3D and placed in situ with a stable, design-compliant fit, (Figures 36,37,38)[34] .

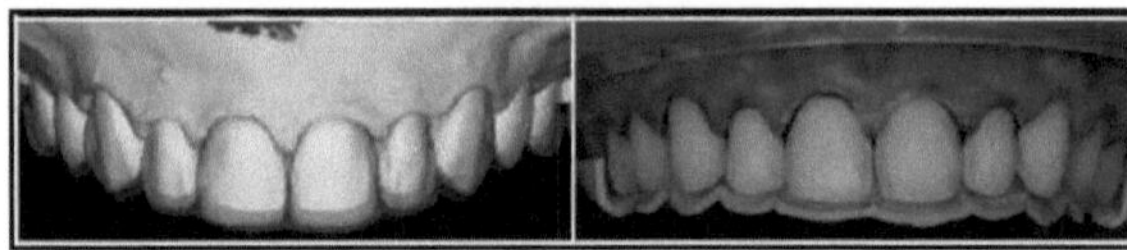

Figure 34: A printed preparation guide for incisal reduction using a digital wax-up[34] .

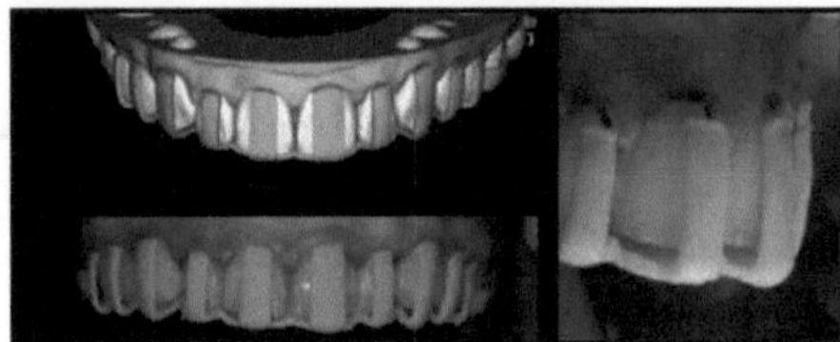

Figure 35: A printed preparation guide for vestibular reduction using the digital wax-up[34] .

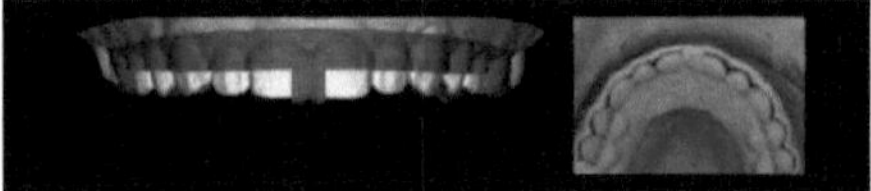

Figure 36:
B: A printed preparation guide for incisal edge reduction using digital wax-up [34]

Digital design allows the practitioner to produce reduction control guides for the vestibular face and incisal edge at the same time.

This design makes it easy to create vertical and horizontal reduction grooves.

Vertical and horizontal windows are created, 3 mm wide and 1 mm deep, with vertical access extending to the incisal edge with an opening of 1.5 mm.

Conservative dental preparations are made using a fine diamond bur, following the vertical and horizontal depth grooves with a 0.5 mm reduction, plus an additional 1.5 mm reduction for the incisal area. The dental reduction guide is then removed and the remaining parts of the tooth are prepared. During this process, the guide should be placed and removed to re-check the amount of tooth structure removed. (Figure 39)[35] .

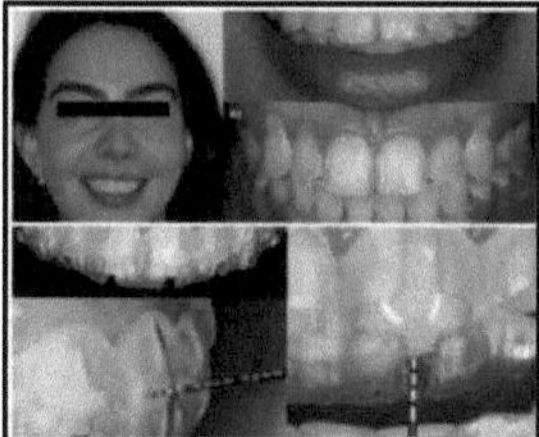

Figure 37: A 3D-printed reduction guide for the vestibular surface and incisal edge. [35]

1.4. First fit kit :

The First Fit system uses 3D-printed guides and a handpiece specially designed for guided veneer preparation. It allows teeth to be reduced to a predetermined depth and area, unlike the use of calibrated burs or silicone guides, which require the process to be interrupted to reassess preparations. (Figure 40 and 41).

Preparation can be carried out in one or two stages.

In the one-step approach, final restorations are produced prior to tooth preparation using reduction guides, and veneers are bonded on the same day as preparation. This approach is indicated when a free-edge/vertical preparation is feasible, as well as in semi-additive cases. This applies in particular to situations where volume can be added in the interproximal and cervical areas, as the system does not allow guided preparation in these areas or precise delineation of the finishing line.

-The two-stage method involves a preparation phase at the first appointment, followed by bonding at the second appointment. In this approach, reduction guides are used to assist incisal and vestibular preparation, and interproximal and cervical preparation is completed freehand ([36]).

In the one-step approach, the number of appointments is reduced. In the two-stage approach, the advantage of the system is that it reduces preparation time for vestibular and incisal surfaces.

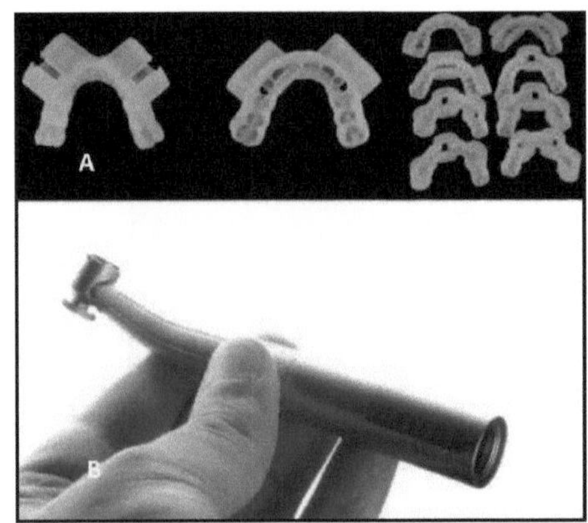

Figure 38: The First Fit system [36]
A: 3D printed guides B: The special First Fit handpiece

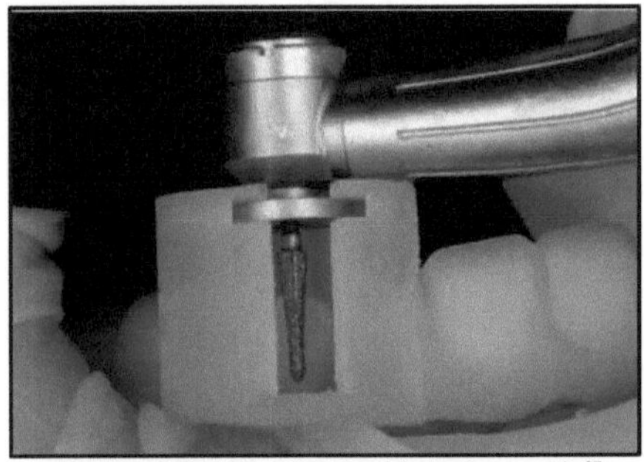

Figure 39:The 3D printed guide in the mouth [37]

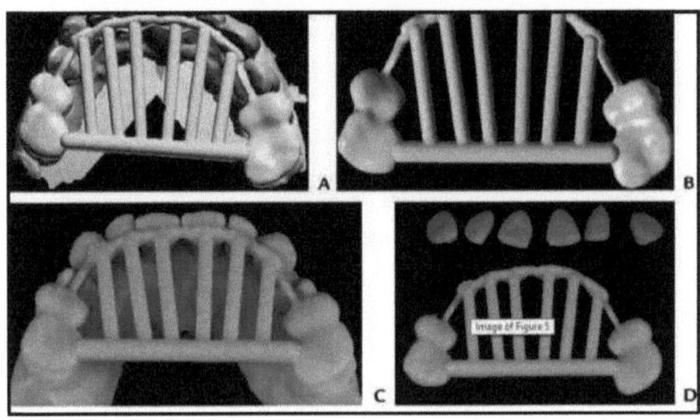

3. The digital footprint

3.1. Optical impression

3.1.1. Definition

For maximum precision and fidelity, and in an attempt to solve all the problems of impression materials, the intra-oral digital scanner system was developed.

From this optical impression, specific software creates a virtual master model, enabling computer-aided design and manufacturing (CAD/CAM).

The 3D preview of dental preparations offers a major advantage by allowing in situ preparation control and brings the necessary rectifications (figures 42 and 43)[38,39]

.

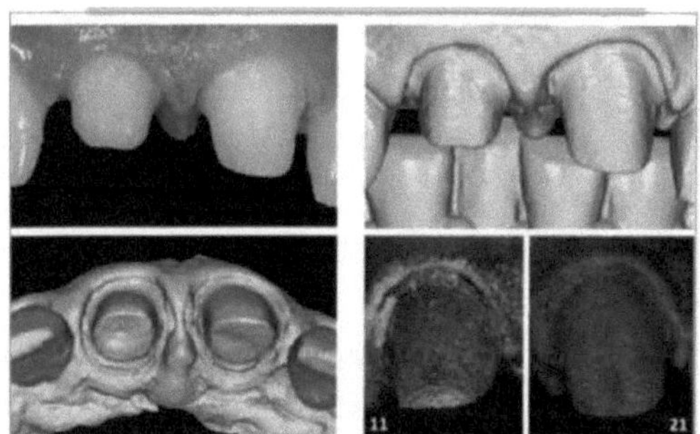

Figure 40: Optical impressions for two prosthetic restorations, 11 and 21. [26]

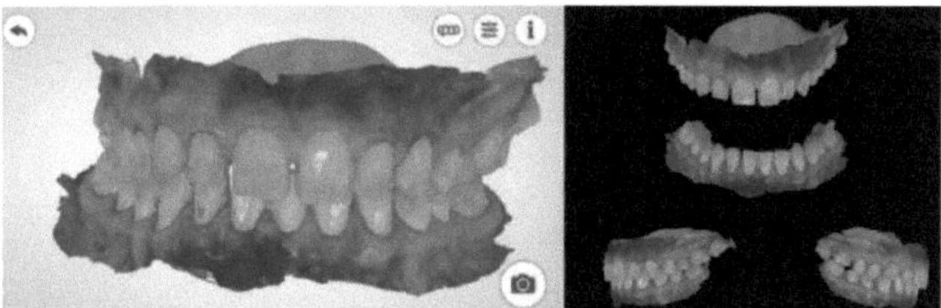

Figure 41: Optical impression of both arches and the right and left intercuspids[37] The first phase of Computer-Aided Design/Manufacturing involves capturing an optical impression using an intra-oral camera,

a step considered essential for reducing inaccuracies, according to Pr François

Duret. This step takes place during direct or semi-direct CAD/CAM acquisition. The choice of impression camera may or may not include the use of a powder system. The acquisition procedure is divided into three stages: firstly, registration of the arcade concerned, then of the antagonist arcade, followed by a vestibular registration of the occlusion in a maximum intercuspid rest position. This first step can be carried out in one or more sessions, and the new digital data is integrated with the existing data. The duration of this digital impression varies according to the practitioner's expertise and the clinical complexity of the case, but with practice it can take between 2 and 5 minutes. (Figure 44 and 45)[26] .

Some devices require the application of a thin layer of matte powder to the surface of the volumes to be recorded. Micronized titanium dioxide was the first material used for this purpose. Its extremely white color makes it easily observable and clearly distinguishable from the oral tissues being recorded.[39]

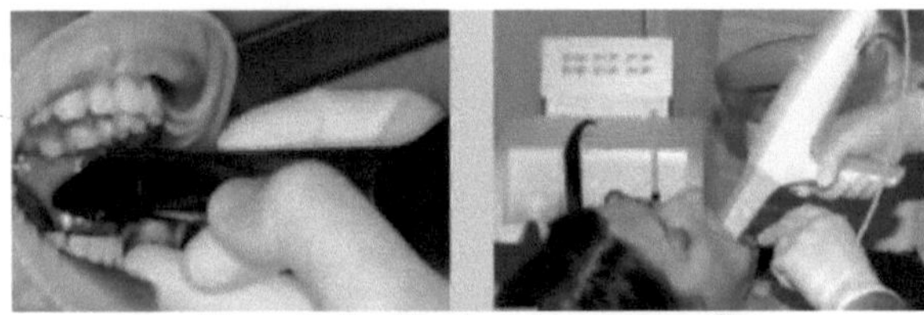

Figure 42: Handling the intraoral camera[39]

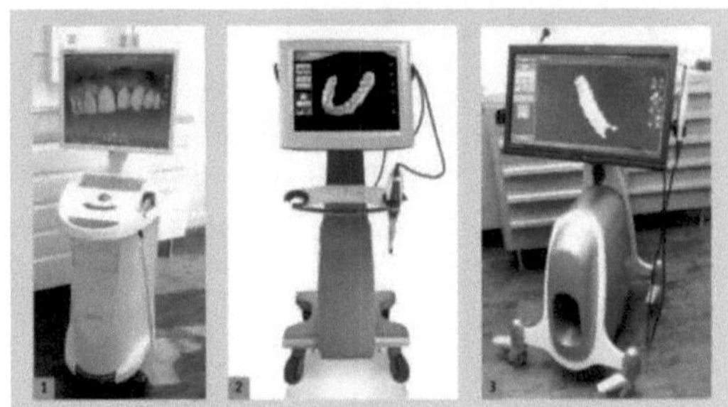

Figure 43:Optical impression systems

This step is generally carried out using :

- Incoherent light emitters (such as lasers), or wave emitters outside the visible light range.
- Specific sensors or receivers for the radiation emitted by the transmitter used.

- Analog/digital converters to decode the analog disturbance transmitted by the sensor and convert it into a digital value.

- Image processing filters that format numerical values into a system that can be understood by computer-aided design (CAD) systems, such as the universal "STL" format.[40]

3.12. Advantages of optical impression

- Accuracy of data obtained
- Unalterable results
- Possibility of completing or correcting the impression at any time
- Elimination of disinfection and packaging steps
- Optimizing communication with the laboratory
- Patient comfort
- Better understanding of the treatment plan by the patient
- Save time and simplify work for the care team [26]

Digital impressions and CAD/CAM technology offer a better marginal fit than those created using conventional techniques(12,55).

According to the study by Yuzbasioglu et al (12), we conclude that :

- The digital impression technique is more efficient than the conventional impression technique. The overall processing time for the conventional impression technique was longer than that for the digital impression technique.
- Digital imprinting is the preferred and most effective technique, according to subject perception.
- The treatment comfort of the digital impression technique is superior to that of the conventional impression technique when performed by an experienced operator.

Research has evaluated the accuracy of conventional and digital impression methods.

The results showed that of the impression systems and materials compared, the best performers were CEREC

And it seems that the precision of digital impressions is on a par with conventional impression methods for veneer fabrication. Both techniques can therefore be used. In conclusion, optical impressions allow better marginal adaptation of veneers (12).

4. Digital color selection tools

All color meters consist of a detector, a signal conditioner and software that processes the signal to make the data more usable in the dental practice or laboratory.

Spectrophotometers, colorimeters and imaging systems have been used to solve visual matching problems. As a result, they improve the accuracy of color readings ,their communication and reproduction in the laboratory, increasing the working efficiency and precision of our aesthetic restorations[44,45].

4.1 Digital cameras and imaging systems

The latest devices used for tooth shade matching are based on digital camera technology.

Instead of focusing light onto a film to create a chemical reaction, digital cameras record images using charge-coupled devices, which comprise thousands or even millions of tiny light-sensitive elements called photosites.

They provide a complete and accurate image of the tooth surface, which is also useful for color mapping. To obtain a full color image, most sensors use filtering to examine light in its three primary colors in an analogous way.

There are several ways of recording the three colors in a digital camera. The highest-quality cameras use three separate sensors, each with a different filter. Light is directed to the different filter/sensor combinations by placing a beam splitter in the camera. The beam splitter allows each sensor to simultaneously view the image[18,46].

4.2 Colorimeter

Colorimeters measure color (hue, luminosity and saturation) as perceived by the human eye under fixed lighting and observation conditions, and filter light in the red, green and blue zones of the visible spectrum. Their main optical elements are the light source, the integrating sphere and the detector (three or four filters). They are considered less accurate than spectrophotometers. Colorimeters do not correspond exactly to the functions of the standard observer, and do not retain adequate sensitivity at low light levels. They measure the quantity of light absorbed globally, whereas spectrophotometers measure the quantity of light absorbed by a specific wavelength (Figure 46)[18/16].

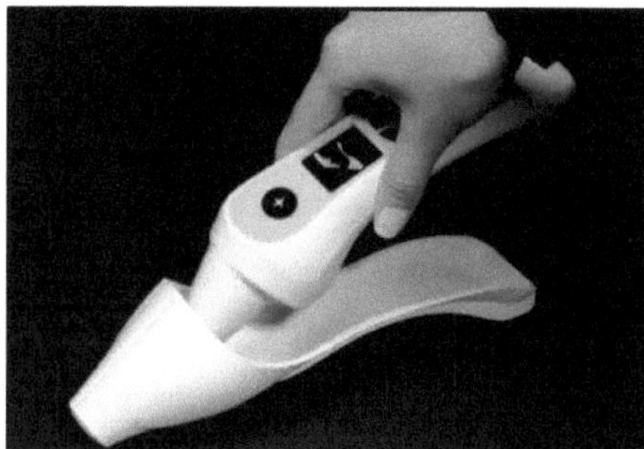

Figure 44: Shade Star colorimeter [47]

4.2.1 Shade vision

It's an imaging colorimeter.

It consists of a portable unit with its own light source, and a liquid crystal display for easy positioning on the tooth.

The complete image of the tooth is provided using three separate databases: the gingiva, the middle third and the incisal third (Figure 47).

The virtual test function enables color reproduction to be tested during production[47].

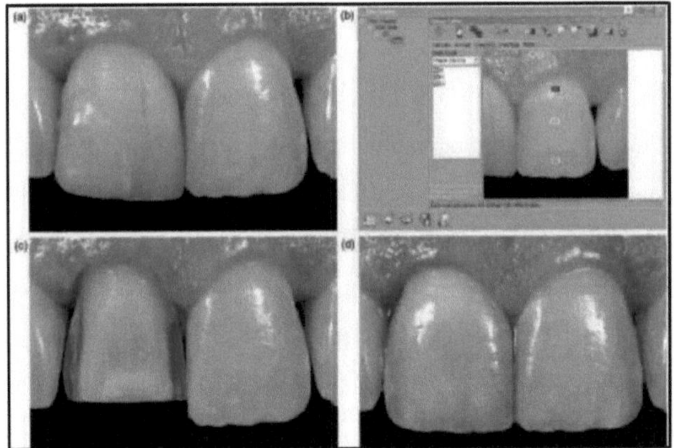

Figure 45: ShadeVision application for facet color selection on 11 [47]

4.3 Spectrophotometer

This is a photometer that measures intensity as a function of color, or more precisely wavelength.

A spectrophotometer contains a source of optical radiation, a means of dispersing the light, a measuring optical system, a detector and a means of converting the light obtained into a signal that can be analyzed.

In general, sources are diffracted, and several wavelengths pass through the input slit and the test sample. The detector converts the intensity of light at a given wavelength into an electrical signal, which is then amplified and displayed on a screen or plotted on a graph.

They measure the amount of light energy reflected by an object at intervals of more than 25 nm along the visible spectrum.

A spectrophotometer is recommended for accurate color measurement. A colorimeter provides an overall measurement of absorbed light, while a spectrophotometer measures light absorbed at different wavelengths. Spectrophotometers are reliable and accurate over time ι≡,i8,46,47.

4.3.1 VITA Easy Shade (VES) intraoral dental spectrophotometer

This is a portable color selection device (Figure 48).

VITA Easy Shade consists of a base unit and a handpiece linked by a fiber-optic cable. The handpiece contains a fiber-optic probe that illuminates and receives light from a tooth, and a microprocessor for communication with the base unit. It illuminates a 5 mm diameter area of the tooth surface.

Before measuring, it is necessary to select a measurement mode (tooth, crown or shade sample)[47].

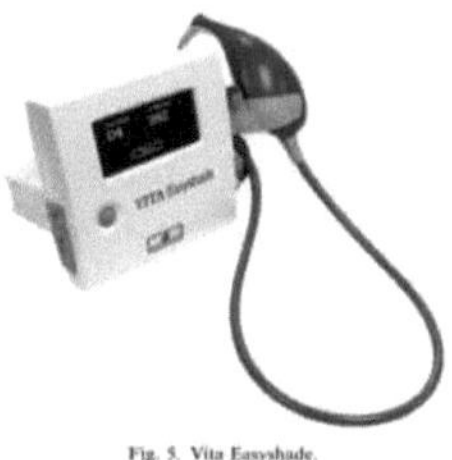

Fig. 5. Vita Easyshade.

Figure 46: EasyShade spectrophotometer [47]

4.3.2. Shade X

Shade-X is also a compact, wireless spectrophotometer for point measurements with a 3 mm diameter probe (Figure 49).

Shade-X uses two databases to match the color of the dentin (more opaque) and the incisal areas of the tooth (more translucent)[47].

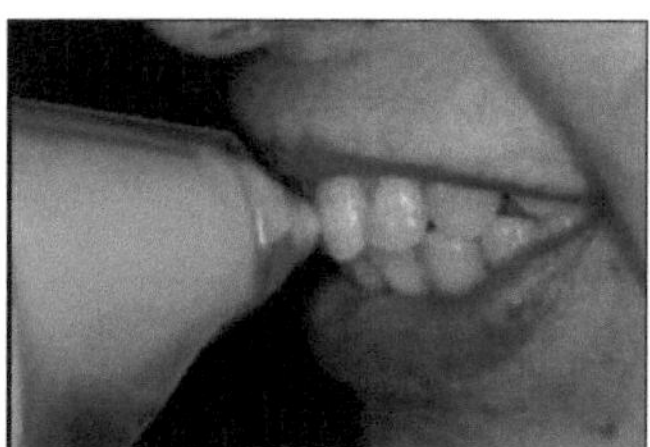

Figure 47: Clinical application of the Shade-X spectrophotometer [47]

4.3.3. Spectroshade micro

This is the most complex dental color imaging spectrophotometer in terms of design and the most cumbersome in terms of hardware. It is the only one to combine digital color imaging with spectrophotometric analysis. The handpiece is relatively large compared to contact probe designs, and positioning can be tricky.

It has an internal computer with analysis software and a guidance system for tooth positioning (Figure 50).

The software contains shade guide references for most ceramic systems, and others can be added.

A digital image of the tooth, shade mapping and colorimetric data can be transmitted electronically or printed to the laboratory.

It provides shade in three distinct zones, cervical, medial and incisal, and gives detailed shade information.
Its virtual verification can be carried out using this system. [47]

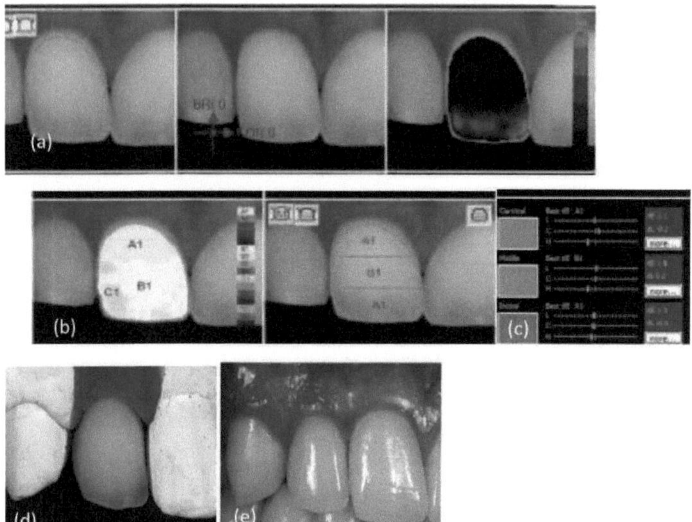

Figure 48: Clinical application of SpectroShade Micro,[47] .

5. Digital bonding aids: optimize bonding precision

One of the factors influencing the marginal adaptation of veneers and their final aesthetic appearance is bonding.

The aesthetic result and durability may be affected if mistakes are made during this phase of the treatment[28] .

5.1. Bonding ceramic veneers using 3D guidance

The bonding of veneers has always been a delicate technique and an arduous task, especially if several veneers are to be fitted at the same time.

The risk of moving, rotating or incorrectly placing veneers up to the finishing line are common clinical problems.
All ceramic partial restorations, and veneers in particular, rely on bonding as a means of retention.

Da Silva et al.[49] in 2021then thought of a 3D printed bonding guide or repositioning key allowing :

1. Maintain veneers after fitting, especially if adjustments are required.
2. Facilitate adhesive protocol on the inner surface of all restorations at the same time.
3. Stabilize restorations during the intraoral bonding process. This technique helps practitioners to facilitate the bonding of ceramic veneers: -Once the veneers have been tried in the mouth, an optical impression is taken and an STL file is generated with the final veneer in place. (Figure 51 and 52).

Based on the digital model of the final veneer, a 3D printed guide is designed(Figure 53)[49] .

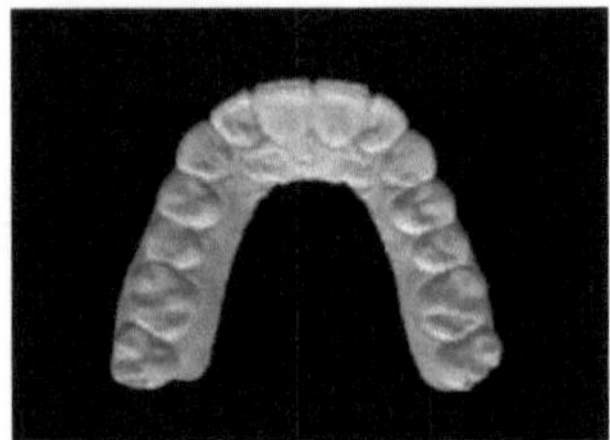

Figure 49: Occlusal view of digital model with veneers in place [49]

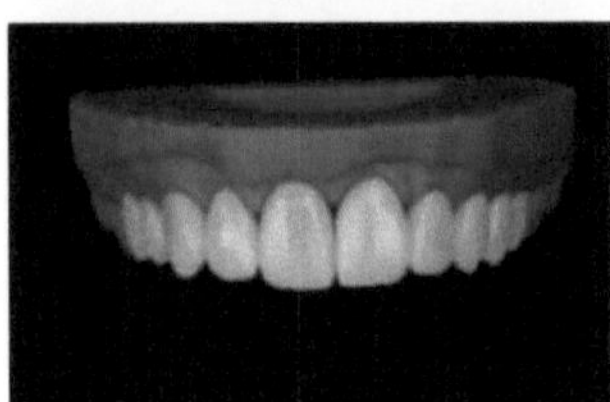

Figure 50: Front view of facets machined on a 3D-printed model

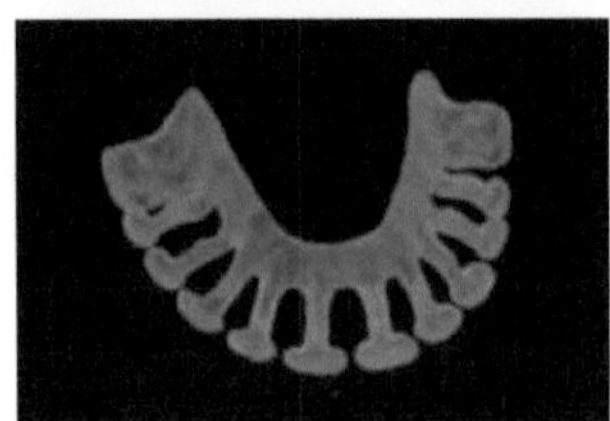

Figure 51: The 3D printed guide

-We ensure that the occlusal and palatal molar supports of all other teeth (Figure 53).

-Individual concave inciso-buccal support extensions were also designed for each veneer to hold them in place after fitting. (Figure 53).

-The guide has been validated and printed with a flexible resin that allows all veneers to be placed individually with different insertion axes.

-We check that the guide fits the printed model with the veneers in place. (Figure 54)

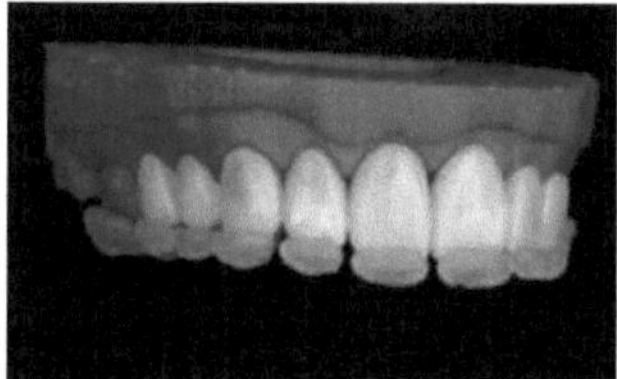

Figure 52: Checking the fit of the 3D-printed tray on the 3D-printed model with the facets in place [49]

The veneers were dry-tried, checking internal fit and interproximal contacts individually.

-Once the veneers were adjusted and the color checked with a trial gel, the 3D-printed guide was placed intraorally to ensure a good fit -The adhesive was applied with a microbrush to the incisal edges of the veneers, the tips of the cúspides and the inner face of the incisal-buccal extensions of the splint.

A small amount of flowable composite resin was applied to the concavity of each inciso-buccal extension of the guide and they were fixed and light-cured for 20 s on the veneers individually, one by one.(Figure 55.)

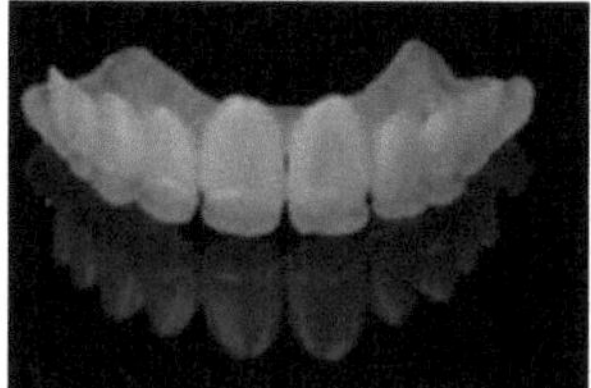

Figure 53: Front view of the veneers bonded to the 3D-printed tray[49]

-The absence of any excess flowable composite resin was confirmed. (Figure 56).

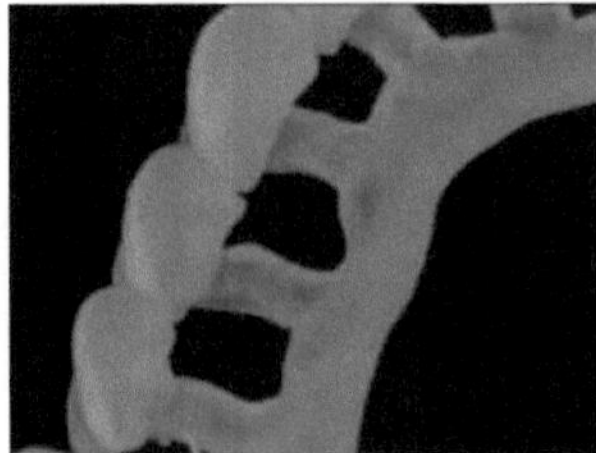

Figure 54: Detailed view to check that no fluid composite resin has penetrated the inner surface of the facets[49]

-Once the veneers have been temporarily bonded to the 3D guide, the inner surfaces of the veneers and the prepared tooth surfaces are treated.

Light-curing resin cement was applied to the inner surface of the veneers and the 3D-printed guide was placed in position, ensuring that the occlusal/palatal rests were correctly adjusted.

-Once in place, each veneer was fitted individually, pressing on the inciso-buccal extension. (Figure 57).

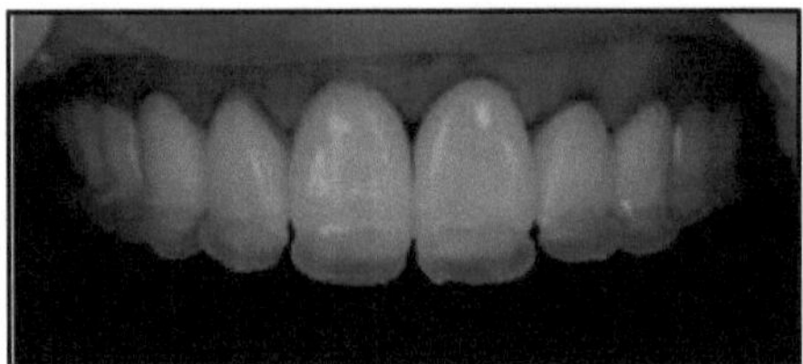

Figure 55: Intraoral front view of 3D-printed tray with veneers ready for adhesive bonding [49]

-All excess cement was removed with a fine micro-brush, and dental floss was used to clean the interproximity.

After a 10-second light-curing of each veneer, the 3D positioning guide was removed to facilitate the palatal surface cleaning process.

-Once the veneers have been bonded, the dam is removed and the occlusion is checked. The silicone key is used to check the thickness and volume of the buccal surface[49] .

Microscopy (from the Greek scopein "to see" and micro "small") is defined as the action of observing objects or entities of very small size, using magnification tools, in particular the microscope, invented in the 16th century by Galileo There are generally two types of magnification tools, also known as optical aids, used in dentistry: magnifying glasses and operating microscopes 50.

1. Definition of optical aids

Optical aids include all devices designed to correct visual deficiencies, prevent or reduce handicaps, or compensate for visual incapacities. They are placed between the operator's eyes and the operating field to facilitate surgery by enlarging the field of vision[51] .

1.1. The concept of magnification

Magnification is divided into three categories:

- Low magnification (3x - 8x)

It is suitable for orienting the tooth and positioning the bur or ultrasonic tip. This level of magnification is used in loupes, which enable simple procedures to be performed competently. (Figure 58 and 59).

- Medium magnification (8x - 16x)

It is commonly used in non-surgical and surgical endodontic procedures, as it offers an acceptable field of view and depth of field. It is used for complex procedures such as perforation repair, recovery of fractured instrument portions and surgical interventions requiring greater precision. (Figure 60).

- High magnification (16x - 30x)

It is mainly used for close-up examinations and tiny anatomical features, such as the calcified orifice of a canal and tiny fissures.

The image below shows the effect of increasing magnification levels, from vision up to x4(Figure 61) (31,23).

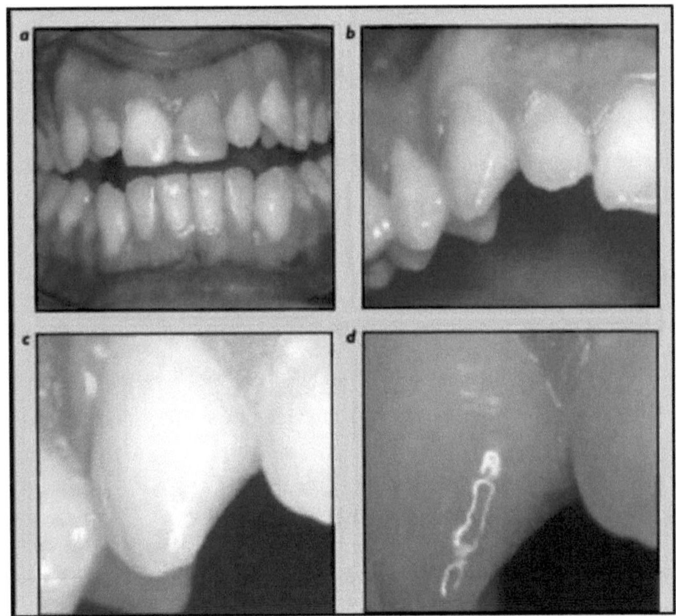

Figure 56: View of the same oral cavity using different magnification powers (23).
a:Without help
b: x2 magnification
c : Magnification x3
d : x4 magnification.

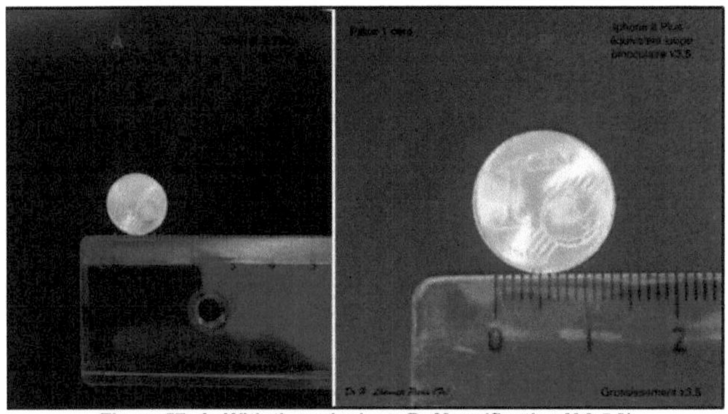

Figure 57: A: With the naked eye B: Magnification X 3.5 [54]

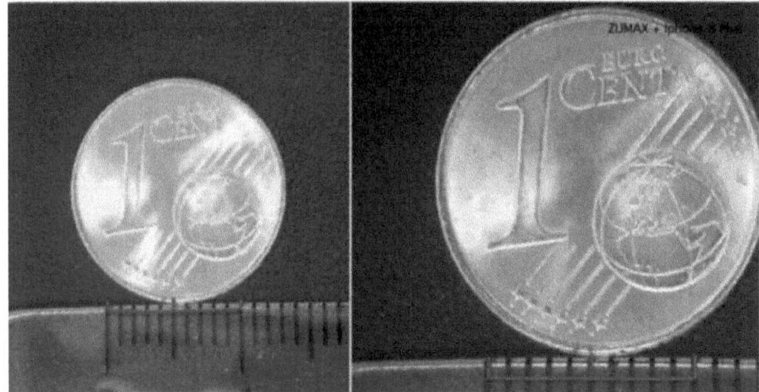

Figure 58: X10 magnification versus X15 magnification [54]

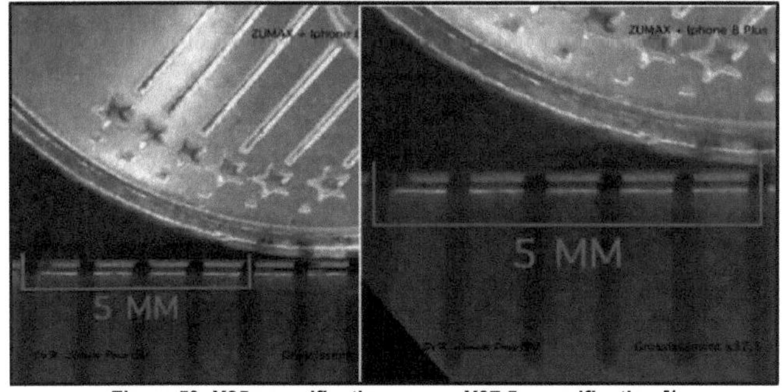

Figure 59: X25 magnification versus X37.5 magnification [54]

2. Operating microscopes

2.1. Definition

The operating microscope is an instrument that enables the operating physician to illuminate and magnify the area to be treated during a surgical procedure, so that all its structures that would otherwise be difficult to observe with the naked eye can be seen with precision.

In dentistry, the operating microscope is an optical instrument that enables the dentist to see a stereoscopic image of the tiny structures at the surgical site. This image is high quality, illuminated and magnified up to 10 times more than with the loupes used by most dentists.

There's no denying that its use enables dental procedures of incomparable precision[9] .

2.2. History

The operating microscope first appeared in medicine, and more particularly in disciplines where microsurgery is performed, such as ophthalmology and neurosurgery.

The first magnification system used in the medical field was developed by the German company Zeiss in the early 1920s. It was a monocular optical microscope with IOx magnification, used in microsurgery by the German Holmegreen. Then came the idea of developing a system for simulating stereoscopic vision (or binocular vision).

In 1953, Zeiss presented the first OPMI 1 stereomicroscope, featuring co-axial illumination and variable working distance.

For many decades, the microscope has been used in various medical and surgical fields, but it was only recently introduced into dentistry, some 40 years ago, by two French dentists, Drs. Boussens and Ducamin (43).

The first true operating microscope in dentistry was developed by Dr. Howard's team at Harvard School (Figure 62).

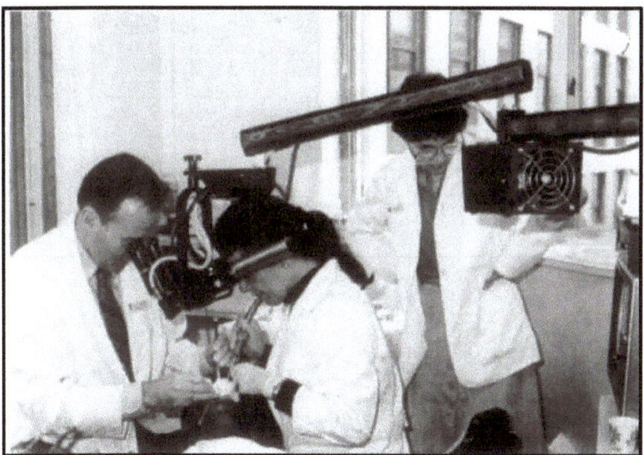

Figure 60: The dentiscope, the first operating microscope in dentistry developed at Havard University: Practitioners work under the dentiscope at X7 magnification, and students watch the procedure live on television.

Its application first began in the field of Tendodontics, then rapidly spread to the fields of oral and periodontal surgery. Recently, restorative and prosthetic dentistry have also been able to benefit from its advantages.

As a result, prosthetic treatments benefit from superior quality, offering significantly greater comfort for both practitioner and patient, and are also more respectful of the environment.

It's all part of the same logic: "You can do what you can see": better vision equals better practice.

Academic institutions, advanced training courses or continuing education sessions even incorporate the microscope as a learning tool.

In fixed prosthetics, laboratory technicians initially used the first stereomicroscope to highlight preparation limits and edge finishing (Figure 63) (1,11).

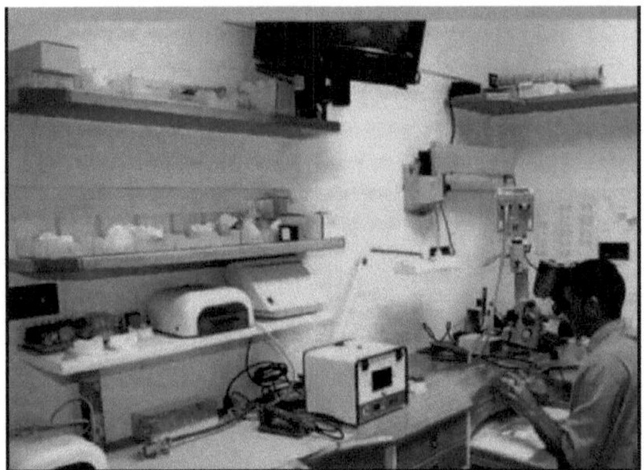

Figure 61: Using the microscope in the prosthetics laboratory [58]

Because of the attention to detail required, the use of enlargement systems in everyday practice continues to grow.

2.3. Microscope components

2.3.1. Optical principle of a microscope

The operating microscope consists of a complex optical system of lenses, offering binocular and stereoscopic vision, with an overall magnification of 4 to 40.

Unlike binocular magnifiers, the two main beams arrive parallel on the observer's retina (Figure 64), so no convergence is required. This results in minimal strain on the eye muscles.

Today's microscopes are designed according to Galilean stereoscopy: in other words, each eye perceives a distinct image of the object through the objective lens[51]

.

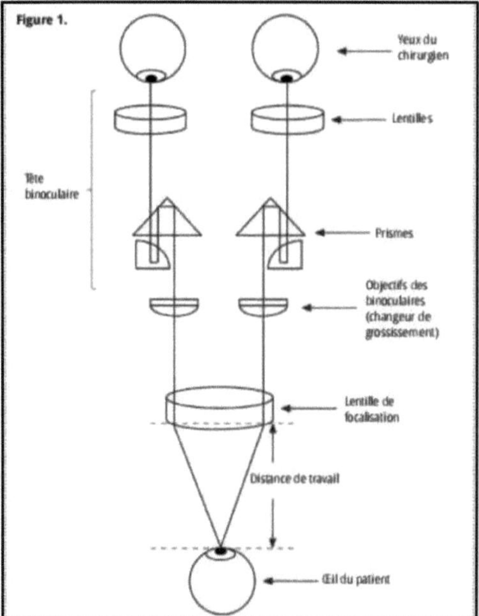

Figure 62: Galilean stereomicroscope [59]

2.3.2. The components

An operating microscope consists of :

2.3.2.1. The eyepiece

The role of the eyepiece is to magnify the image formed in the binocular tube. Eyepieces are available with magnifications of 10x, 12.5x, 16x and 20x.

When choosing an eyepiece, not only the magnification, but also the size of the operating field is important.

Modern eyepieces offer the possibility of correcting abnormalities in the operator's vision within a range of -8 to +8 dioptres. This correction only concerns convergence anomalies, and glasses are still required for astigmatism (Figure 65) (9,19,33,).

2.3.2.2. The binocular tube

There are two types of tube: straight and angled.

Straight tubes allow observation parallel to the microscope axis, while angled tubes allow observation at 45 degrees to the axis.

There are adjustable-tube microscopes, also known as binocular tubes, with steplessly adjustable viewing angles.

In dentistry, for ergonomic reasons, only the swivel tube is considered, offering angle adjustment from 0° to 180° without a stop (Figure 65)[51] .

2.3.1.1. The objective

This is used to project the light from the illumination source onto the operating field, thanks to two successive deflections by prisms, creating coaxial illumination.

Its purpose is to focus light rays. In dentistry, 20 cm lenses are generally recommended (Figure 65)[51] .

2.3.1.2. Demonstration or observation eyepiece

It is possible to have a demonstration eyepiece and a secondary observation tube. This allows 1 or 2 secondary observers to follow the examination or procedure without disturbing the stereoscopic vision of the primary observer (Figure 65) 5i.

2.3.1.3. The magnification changer

Also known as the "Galileo changer", it consists of a cylinder containing a system of two telescopes, each comprising a converging and a diverging lens, offering different magnification factors.

By combining the magnification selector with the corresponding objectives and eyepieces, it is possible to obtain an increasing series of magnifications from 0.5 to 2.5 by simply rotating the roller.

This function can be activated either by a foot pedal or by a manual rotary switch located on the microscope housing (Figure 65)[51] .

2.3.1.4. Lighting system

A major advantage of the operating microscope is its illumination system. Operating microscopes are fitted with cold-light mirrors that eliminate infrared rays. This heat radiation could unexpectedly heat up the surgical field.
In an ophthalmic microscope, the light is generally coaxial and follows the same path as the image to prevent shadows[51] .

2.3.1.5. The distance

The working distance is the distance between the focusing lens and the focal point of the optical system. This fixed value is determined by the focal length of the selected focusing lens. Its choice depends on the type of operation
Precise adjustment of the user's inter-pupillary distance is essential to ensure adequate stereoscopic vision of the operating field[59] .

2.3.1.6. The stand

An operating microscope is a bulky piece of equipment. Its configuration can vary according to the layout of the dental practice, to make it as ergonomic as possible for the dentist.
It can be mounted on a base, or preferably suspended from the ceiling like the operating light, or wall-mounted. Here, the ProErgo model, from Zeiss, has advanced features, making it more convenient to use (variable focus, electromagnetic brakes controlled by a simple touch of the finger to assist head movement, high-intensity light, etc.). (Figure 66) (19, 61).

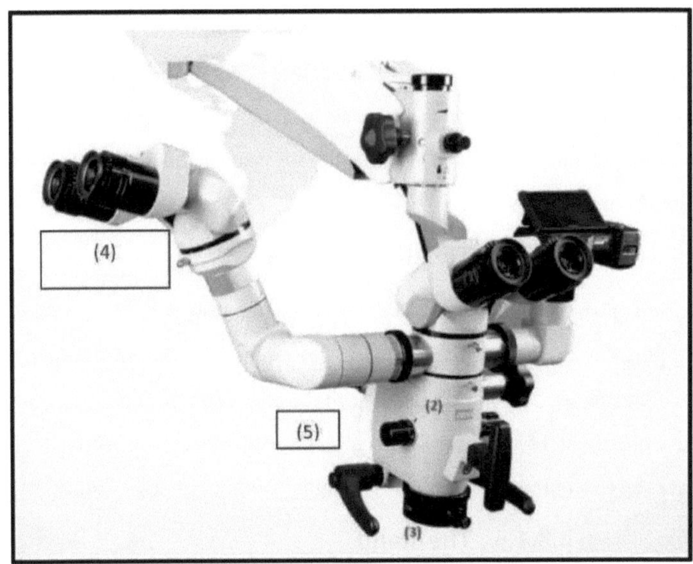

Figure 63: Operating microscope components
1 :the eyepiece,2 :the binocular tube,3 :the objective,4 :demonstration or observation eyepiece,5 :the magnification changer [59]

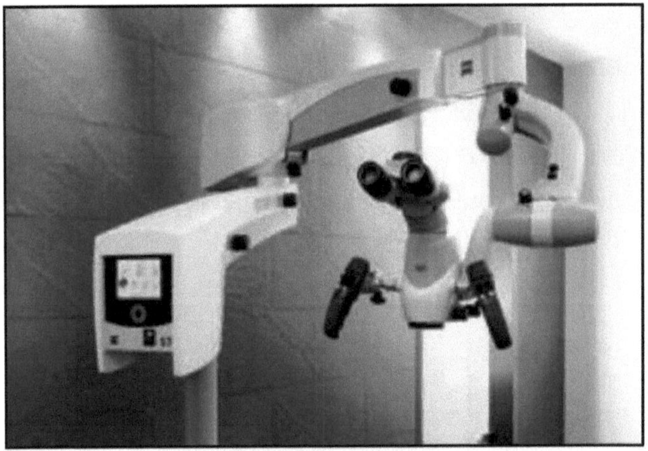

Figure 64: Zeiss ProErgo operating microscope [59]

- Mobile stand :

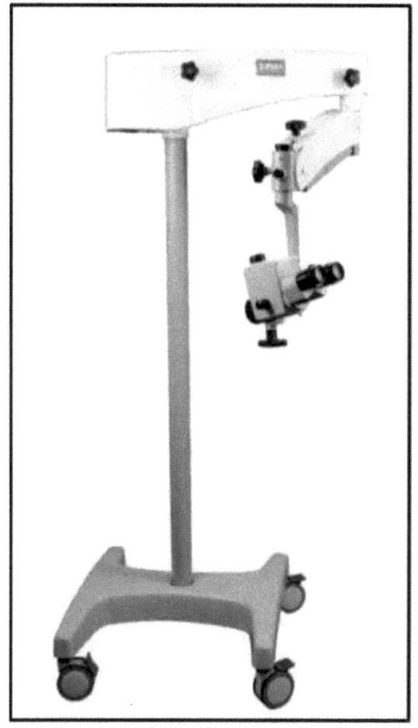

Figure 65: Zumax OMS 2350 dental operating microscope [61]

- Wall-mounted stand

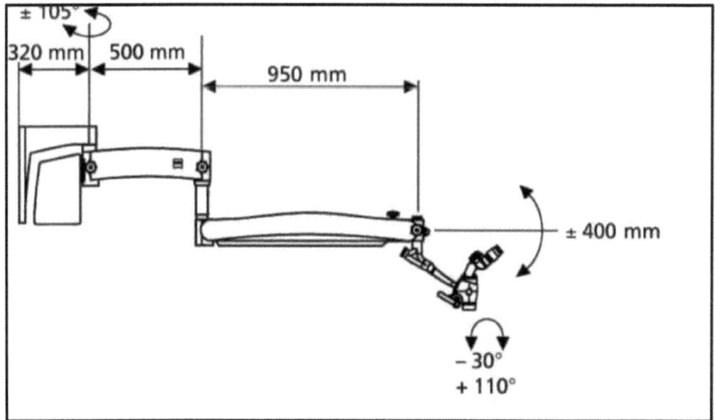

Figure 66: Wall-mounted stand [62]

- Ceiling-mounted stand

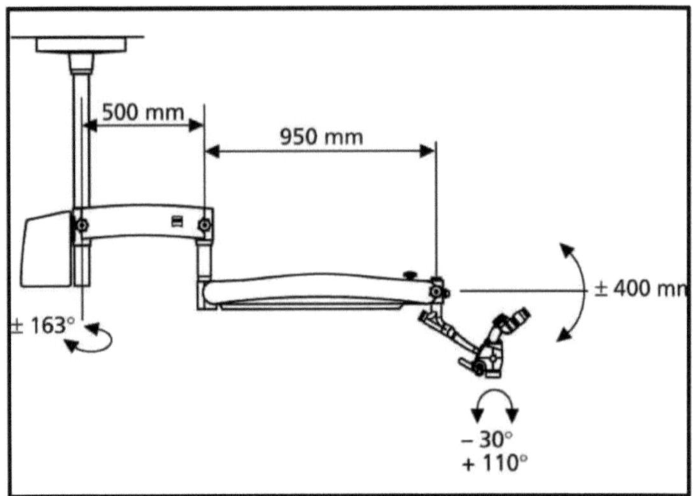

Figure 67: Ceiling-mounted stand [62]

The latter two configurations take up minimal space compared with the former.

2.4. The features you need in a microscope

The ideal clinical microscope for restoration can have many variations, but several essential features are necessary:

- Stable mounting: The stability of the microscope is an important feature that helps avoid micromovements of the instrument, which disrupt the operator's visual image during use.
- An arm long enough to comfortably extend the distance between the focusing lens and the operating field.
- Excellent optics with multiple magnifications available: these variable magnification levels offer the practitioner unlimited flexibility to optimize visual acuity in all clinical situations, as well as precise focusing, coaxial illumination and light shields.

- Ideally, the microscope should be positioned to the left of the patient for right-handed users, and approximately at hip level.
- Adjustment capability: This not only allows greater flexibility in the vertical dimension, but also enables the microscope body to be positioned on several axes, while maintaining a comfortable position for the binocular eyes.
- The presence of a light-curing filter is useful for restorative applications of light-sensitive materials under microscope-assisted vision during adhesion and bonding procedures. The filter enables the dentist to view the field with adequate light on light-sensitive composite materials without the frustration of premature curing.
- For practitioners wishing to document procedures, audiovisual media offer an ideal configuration for documentation across the field of vision.
- The microscope allows work to be carried out in a variety of positions, without compromising the ergonomics of the operator. With the microscope, the dentist can adopt a totally physiological posture, with the head vertical to the spine, for optimum comfort. Indeed, when working with the microscope, the dentist looks straight ahead, rather than at the operating field, and can thus maintain an upright posture, eliminating any non-physiological curves in the spine (8, 43,47).

2.5. The advantages of optical microscopy for ceramic veneers

- More precise adaptation of the facets (Figure 70).
- Reduced mental and physical strain for practitioners.
- Controlling the amount of reduction during tooth preparation and minimizing dentine exposure, especially in the case of ceramic veneers.
- Improved lighting power eliminates all blind spots in the field of vision, avoiding the problem of shadows, and enabling better perception of details.
- The ability to document clinical procedures. In fact, most operating microscopes

can be fitted with a camera or cell phone, making it possible to record operating procedures. (Figure 71).

- Improving overall treatment quality.
- The dentist's comfort and motivation.
- Avoiding iatrogenic damage allows the dentist to be extremely precise in his movements while using aggressive rotary instruments.
- Ease of observing the horizontal marginal space between dentures and abutments [2,5,14,50,64]

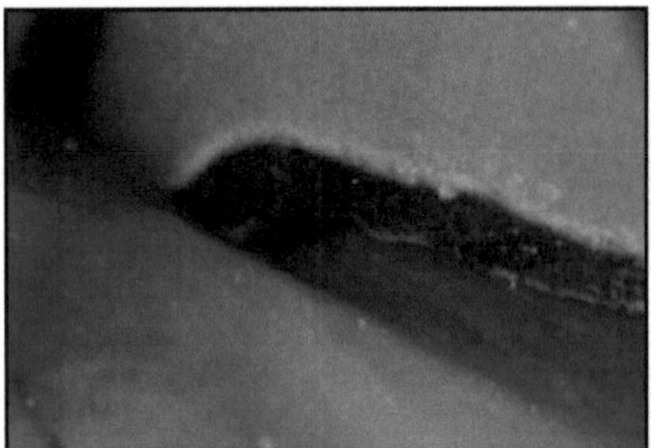

Figure 68:During a fitting session, excessive marginal space between the crown and the tooth can be observed under the microscope and instantly documented. [50]

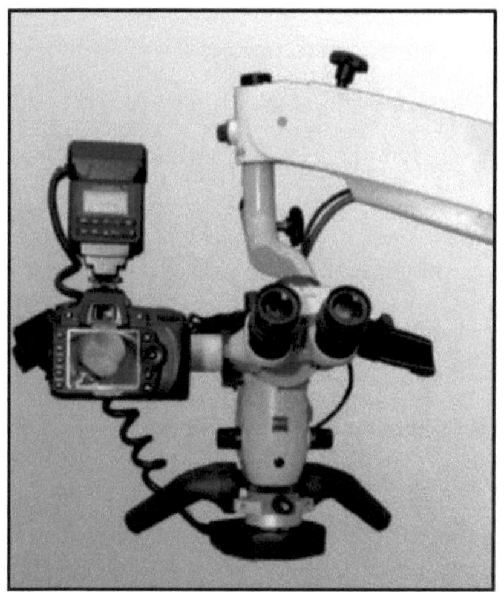

Figure 69: A Nikon D90 microscope and a Sigma Ring Flash for a Zeiss Pico microscope [50]

2.6. The limits of the optical microscope

Limitations include the high cost of this equipment and the specific training required to use it.

The limited field of view at high magnification can also be seen as a disadvantage for some procedures, as focus and area of interest are easily lost during patient movement.

The most important point is that there must be a measurable three-dimensional (3D) reference system beneath the microscopic field of view[64] .

2.7. Microscope maintenance

- It's important to keep the microscope in a cool, dry, well-ventilated place to prevent fungus growth on optics such as lenses.
- We recommend cleaning the optics once a week, following the instructions for cleaning optical surfaces.

- A dust cover is recommended to protect the microscope from dust when not in use. Vinyl covers are preferable, as they are lint-free, unlike cloth covers. However, they should not be used in humid environments, as they can retain moisture, increasing the risk of fungus formation.
- External surfaces should be cleaned with a damp cloth dipped in hot soapy water.
- The foot pedal must be covered with a transparent plastic bag or cover to prevent surgical fluids and cleaning products from damaging its electronic components.
- Before using the microscope, check that the suspension arm can be held in place to ensure that it does not fall on the patient[59] .

3. Magnifiers

These are the most commonly used magnification systems in dentistry. They offer variable magnification from 1.5x to IOx.

Magnifiers have a number of features in common:

- One degree of magnification.
- Binocular vision with optics converging towards the focal length.
- The need for the operator's eyes to converge and adapt[56] .

3.1. Optical principles of magnifiers

There are a number of optical principles specifically related to loupes that are important for the practitioner

- The field of vision
- Depth of field
- The declination or observation angle (figure 72)[65] .

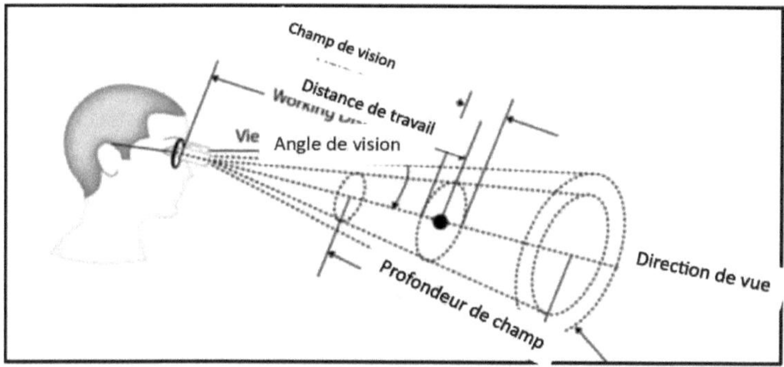

Figure 70: Optical terminology[65]

- Field of vision:

Field width is the size of the operating area when viewed through magnifiers. It is related to telescope diameter, optical design, lens distance, eye and magnification power. The higher the power, the smaller the field[66] .

- Depth of field :

Depth of field refers to the ability of the lens system to maintain focus on near and distant objects without having to change position. As magnification increases, the depth of field decreases, to the point where only a small part of the object can be in focus[65] .

Declination angle :

This is the angle at which a lens is positioned in relation to a horizontal reference line running from the upper loop of the ear to the bridge of the nose, and determines the line of vision. In use, the greater the angle to this line, the greater the neck tilt required to see the object.

From an ergonomic point of view, it is essential to ensure that this angle is correct, to minimize strain on the neck, back and shoulders[65] .

3.2. The different types of magnifiers

The different types of loupes used in dentistry :

- Simple magnifiers :
- Galilean magnifiers,

- Keplerian magnifiers[50] .

3.2.1. Simple magnifiers or spectacle magnifiers

The spectacle magnifier is the simplest and most economical type of magnifier. This type of magnification is an extension of reading glasses, which are actually low-power spectacles. They have the advantage of being cheaper and easier to use, but their magnification power is limited. These magnifiers use a simple magnification system close to the eye subject to aberration.

For optical reasons, the distance to the object decreases with increasing magnification (Figure 73,74,75)[53 ,67] .

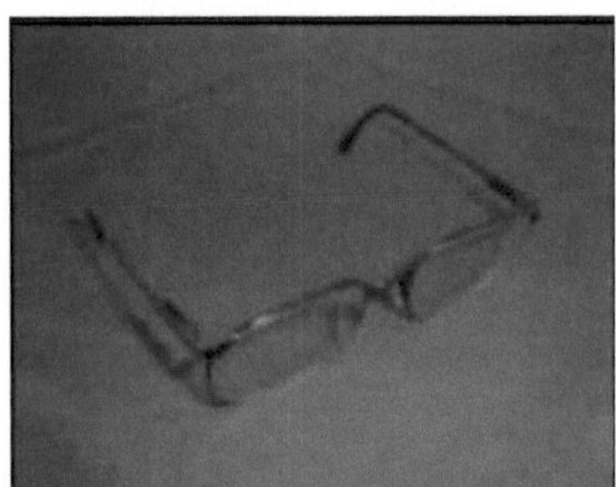

Figure 71: Single magnifier in spectacle frames [53]

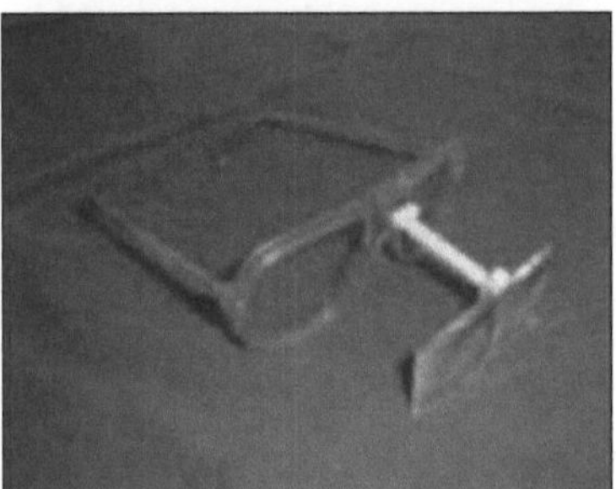

Figure 72: Magnifying glass attached to telescope frame [53]

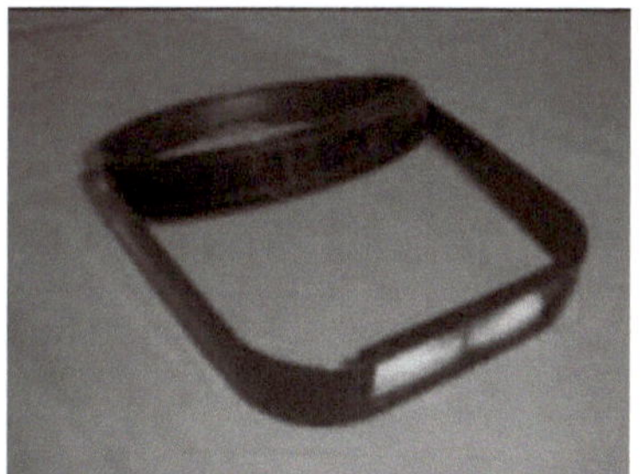

Figure 73: Magnifying glass attached to a headband [53]

3.2.2. Galilean magnifiers

Also known as Galilean telescopic loupes (figure 76 and 77) Galilean loupes are the most common type of magnifier used in dentistry. They have a typical conical shape The Galilean telescope consists of two lenses: a concave eyepiece and a convex objective.

Principle :

The optical principle of Galileo's telescope is to produce an effect similar to that of a thick magnifying glass.

The optical system consists of a combination of convex and concave lenses, whose working distance can be adjusted to suit ergonomic requirements. The eye receives image-forming light beams, which pass through the peripheral zones of the Galilean system, causing distortion and aberration. (Figure 78).

Although the magnification factor is physically limited to 2.5×, it is possible to achieve higher magnification, up to 3.5×, but with optical compromises (limited field of view, blurred edges).

Another point to bear in mind is that all Galilean lens systems produce a halo effect at the periphery of the visual field which, in some cases, can be annoying (Figure 71and 72) [60,65,67].

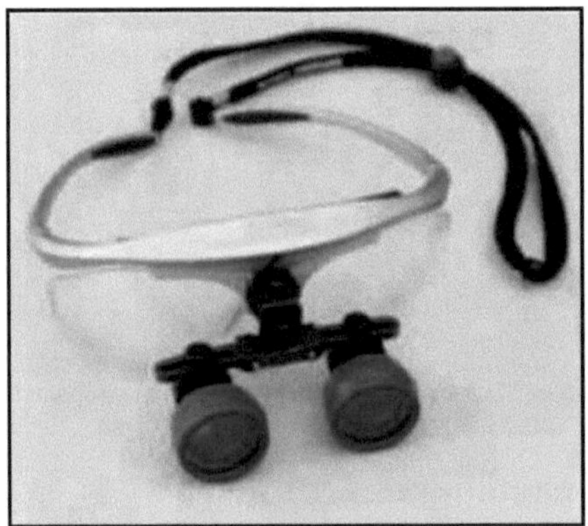

Figure 74: Galilean magnifier [65]

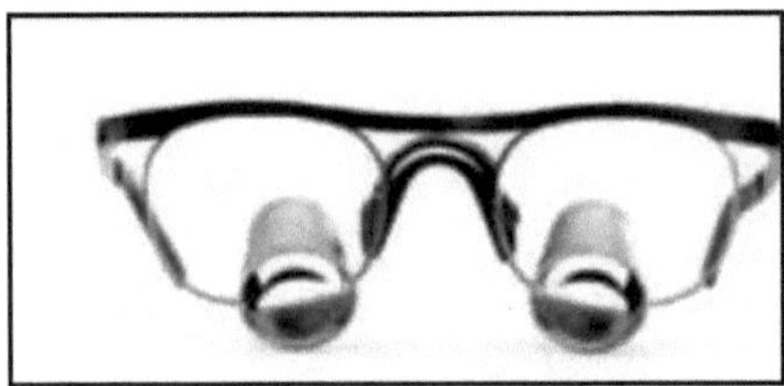

Figure 75: Galilean magnifier through lenses [65]

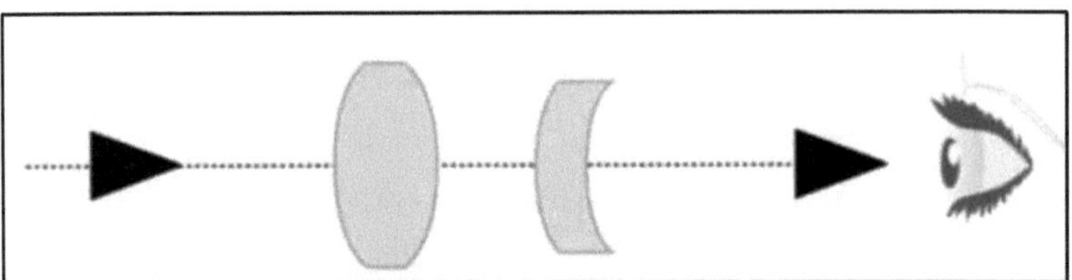

Figure 76: Galilean magnifier principle [65]

3.2.3. Keplerian prism magnifiers

Principle: In Kepler's optical system, the optical principle is such that the main ray always passes through the center of the lens, forming a real diaphragm in the field of view where aberrations are barely perceptible. (Figure 79). These magnifiers are made up of several convergent lenses and can be used to obtain different magnifications and working distances. They offer a good compromise between magnification and depth of field, as well as width and angle of binocular convergence. They are essential for relaxed stereoscopic vision.

These magnifiers provide better magnification quality, wider fields of view and greater depth of field. They can be used for all magnification levels.

Keplerian magnifiers are the most powerful, and a helmet helps to reduce the discomfort generated by their heavy weight and long optics. The disadvantages are that they are heavier, have long barrels and are more expensive (Figure 80) (1,19, 28, 50).

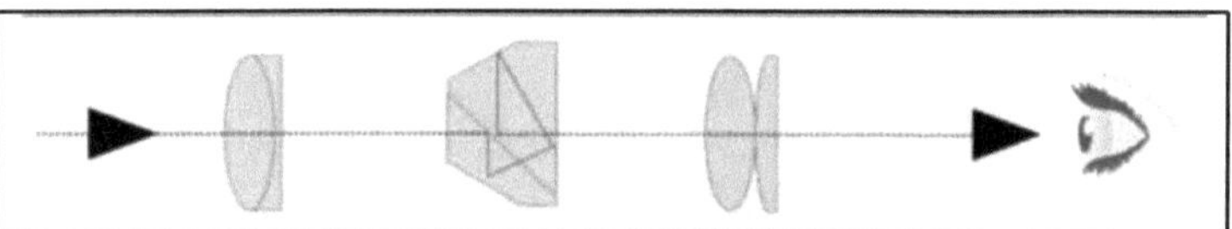

Figure 77: Principle of Keplerian magnifiers [65]

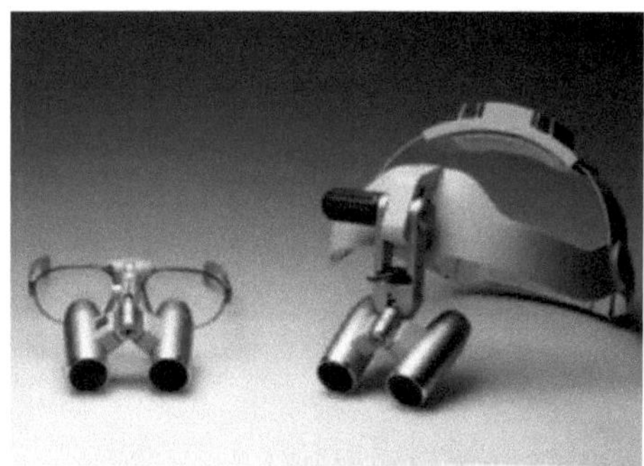

Figure 78: Keplerian magnifiers [65]

3.3. Galilean or Keplerian magnifiers?

When choosing a magnifier, there's always a trade-off between optics and ergonomics. A bright, highly magnified image means extra weight, less depth of field and a limited field of vision. Overall, the use of magnifiers has improved visual acuity. Keplerian magnifiers were far superior to Galilean magnifiers. In all age groups, they deliver significantly better detail detection, with an increase of up to 200% to 400% compared with the naked eye. This is due, on the one hand, to the higher magnification factor and, on the other, to the superior optical properties of Keplerian magnifiers compared with Galilean systems. Galilean loupes offer mainly ergonomic advantages for practitioners, while they can almost completely compensate for presbyopia in the ≥40 years age group (Figure 81 and 82)[67] .

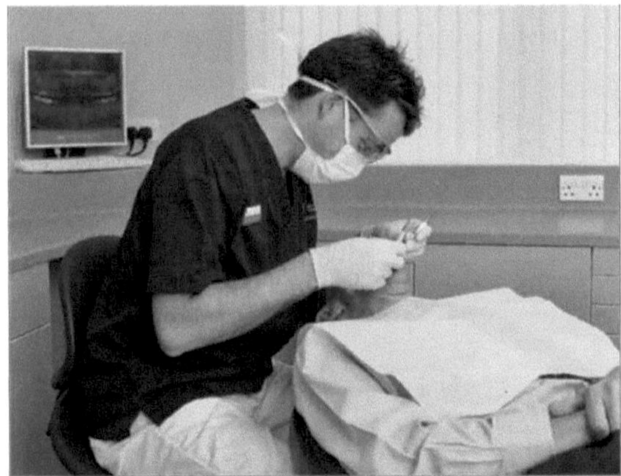
Figure 79: Posture without optical aid[68]

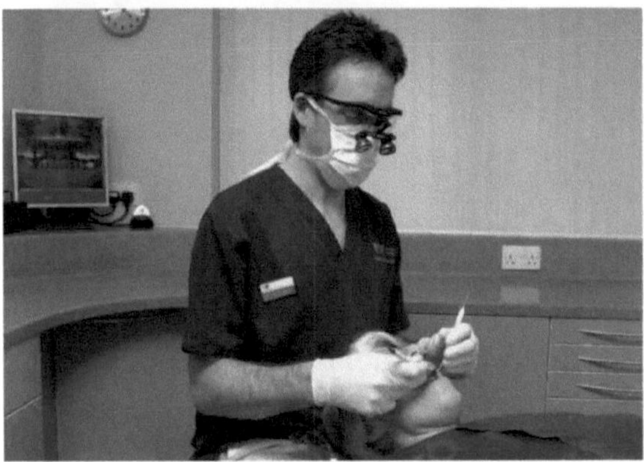
Figure 80: Posture with optical aid [68]

3.4. Advantages over the operating microscope

- Dental magnifiers are less expensive than operating microscopes.
- Easy to use without major image modification[64] .

3.5. Disadvantages

- Magnifiers offer convergent visibility: The two optics of magnifiers have their long axis converging towards a point corresponding to the focal length. As a result, the eyes have to follow the same path and adapt, leading to eye fatigue over prolonged use. This induces stress on the oblique and right medial muscles of the eyeball, as well as on the ciliary muscles of the cornea.
- Magnifiers offer a single magnification, lower than that provided by the clinical microscope.
- With the gaze always directed towards the operating field, the operator is subjected to non-physiological curvatures of the spine, particularly at the cervical level, and must activate numerous paravertebral muscles to maintain this posture.
- Magnifiers cannot provide light. This light is only possible if supplemented by an illumination system. This increases their cost and weight and is detrimental to patient comfort[2,50].

Conclusion

Ceramic veneers represent a reliable and durable aesthetic treatment option, thanks to significant advances in the field over the last twenty years. These advances have significantly improved the durability, aesthetics and reliability of ceramic veneers, offering patients high-quality aesthetic and functional solutions. The use of optical aids improves the precision and quality of veneering procedures, enabling dentists to carry out more predictable treatments. The practitioner's precision is considerably enhanced thanks to an optimal view of the surgical field, which increases the success rate and ensures that patients benefit from outstanding aesthetic results while preserving their natural tooth structure and a beautiful, permanent smile. Improved optical aids, light sources and the emergence of auto-focusing devices are making dentistry in general, and the successful creation of ceramic veneers in particular, even easier, but the optimal use of digital and microscopic tools requires a certain amount of training and in-depth knowledge on the part of the practitioner. Training in this field is still necessary to improve the treatment of veneers as a delicate technique and an arduous task[10 42 65 69] .

References

1. **Aboalshamat K, Daoud O, Mahmoud LA et al.**
   Practices and attitudes of dental loupes and their relationship to musculoskeletal disorders among dental practitioners.
   Int J Dent 2020;2020:1 -7.
2. **ALGhazali N, Laukner J, Burnside G, Jarad FD, Smith PW, Preston AJ.**
   An investigation into the effect of try-in pastes, uncured and cured resin cements on the overall color of ceramic veneer restorations: An in vitro study.
   J Dent 2010;38:78-86.
3. **AlSaleh S, Labban M, AlHariri M, Tashkandi E.**
   Evaluation of self shade matching ability of dental students using visual and instrumental means.
   J Dent 2012;40:82-7.
4. **Bergen SF, McCasland J.**
   Dental operatory lighting and tooth color discrimination.
   J Am Dent Assoc 1977;94:130-4.
5. **Borse S, Chaware S.**
   Tooth shade analysis and selection in prosthodontics: A systematic review and meta-analysis.
   J Indian ProsthodontSoc 2020;20:131 -40.
6. **Brewer JD, Wee A, Seghi R.**
   Advances in color matching.
   Dent CHn North Am 2004;48:341-58.
7. **Bud MG, Pop OD, Cîmpean S.**
   Benefits of using magnification in dental specialties - a narrative review.
   Med Pharm Rep 2023;96:254-7.
8. **Bud M, Jitaru S, Lucaciu O et al.**
   The advantages of the dental operative microscope in restorative dentistry.
   Med Pharm Rep 2020;9(1):1-6.
9. **Burkhardt R.**

New directions in periodontal plastic surgery.

Mens Swiss Med Dent 1999;109:650-5.

10. **Caponi L, Raslan F, Roig M.**

Fabrication of a facially generated tooth reduction guide for minimally invasive preparations: A dental technique.

J Prosthet Dent 2022;127:689-94.

11. **Carr GB.**

Microscopes in endodontics.

J Calif Dent Assoc 1992;20:55-61.

12. **Carvalho TF, Lima JFM, De-Matos JDM et al.**

Evaluation of the accuracy of conventional and digital methods of obtaining dental impressions.

IntJ Odontostomatol 2018;12:368-75.

13. **Cazier S, Moussally C.**

Description of the various digital impression systems.

Rev OdontStomat 2013;42:107-18.

14. **Cho SH, Nagy WW.**

Labial reduction guide for laminate veneer preparation.

J Prosthet Dent 2015;114:490-2.

15. **Christensen GJ.**

Will digital impressions eliminate the current problems with conventional impressions?

JAm DentAssoc 2008;139:761-3.

16. **Chu SJ, Trushkowsky RD, Paravina RD.**

Dental color matching instruments and systems. Review of clinical and research aspects.

J Dent 2010;38:2-16.

17. **Cicciù M, Fiorillo L, D'Amico C et al.**

3D digital impression systems compared with traditional techniques in dentistry: A recent data systematic review.

Materials 2020;13(8):1-18.

18. **Corcodel N, Helling S, Rammelsberg P, Hassel AJ.**

Metameric effect between natural teeth and the shade tabs of a shade guide.

Eur J Oral Sci 2010;118:311-6.

19. **Cordero I.**

Understanding and maintaining an operating microscope.

Rev Sante OculaireComm 2016;13:20-1.

20. **Derbabian K, Marzola R, Donovan TE, Arcidiacono A.**

The science of communicating the art of esthetic dentistry. Part III: Precise shade communication.

J Esthet Restor Dent 2001;13:154-62.

21. **El-Mowafy O, El-Aawar N, El-Mowafy N.**

Porcelain veneers: An update.

Dent Med Probl 2018;55:207-11.

22. **Etienne O, Hajtò J.**

Ceramic materials in metal-free prosthetics.

Cah Prothèse 2011;155:5-13.

23. **Forgie AH.**

Magnification: What is available, and will it aid your clinical practice?

Dent Update 2001;28:125-30.

24. **Gracis S, Thompson V, Ferencz J, Silva N, Bonfante E.**

A new classification system for all-ceramic and ceramic-like restorative materials.

IntJ Prosthodont 2016;28:227-35.

25. **Haddad HJ, Jakstat HA, Arnetzl G et al.**

Does gender and experience influence shade matching quality?

J Dent 2009;37:40-4.

26. **Hamlett K.**

The art of veneer cementation.

Alpha Omegan 2009;102:128-32.

27. **Hampé-Kautz V, Salehi A, Senger B, Etienne O.**

A comparative in vivo study of new shade matching procedures.

IntJ Comput Dent 2020;23:317-23.

28. **James T, Gilmour AS.**

Magnifying loupes in modern dental practice: An update.

Dent Update 2010;37:633-6.

29. **Juggins KJ.**

Current products and practice: The bigger the better: Can magnification aid orthodontic clinical practice?

J Orthod 2006;33:62-6.

30. **Liberato WF, Barreto IC, Costa PP, De Almeida CC, Pimentel W, Tiossi R.**

A comparison between visual, intraoral scanner, and spectrophotometer shade matching: A clinical study.

J Prosthet Dent 2019;121:271-5.

31. **Low JF, Dom TN, Baharin SA.**

Magnification in endodontics: A review of its application and acceptance among dental practitioners.

Eur J Dent 2018;12:610-6.

32. **Magne P, Belser UC.**

Novel porcelain laminate preparation approach driven by a diagnostic mockup.

J Esthet Restor Dent 2004;16:7-16.

33. **Mamoun J, Wilkinson ME, Feinbloom R.**

Technical aspects and clinical usage Ofkeplerian and galilean binocular surgical loupe telescopes used in dentistry or medicine.

Surg Dent Ergonomic Loupes 2013;10(2):1-11.

34. **Marques S, Ribeiro P, Gama C, Herrero-Climent M.**

Digital guided veneer preparation: A dental technique.

J Prosthet Dent 2022;4(2):1 -6.

35. **Massironi D, Pascetta R, Romeo G.**

Precision in dental esthetics.

London: Quintessence Publishing, 2006.

36. **Mohammed AO, Mohammed GS, Mathew M, Alzarea B, Bandela V.**

Shade selection in esthetic dentistry: A review.

Cureus 2022;14(3):1-5.

37. **Ng J, Ruse D, Wyatt C.**

A comparison of the marginal fit of crowns fabricated with digital and conventional methods.

J Prosthet Dent 2014;112:555-60.

38. **Konate NY, Pesson DM, Kouame KA et al.**

The benefits of wax-up in the design of a complex fixed prosthetic restoration.

Rev Iv Odonto Stomatol 2017;19(1):33-8.

39. **Paravina RD.**

Performance assessment of dental shade guides.

J Dent 2009;37:15-20.

40. **Pascotto RC, Benetti AR.**

The clinical microscope and direct composite veneer.

Oper Dent 2010;35:246-9.

41. **Peng M, Li C, Huang C, Liang S.**

Digital technologies to facilitate minimally invasive rehabilitation of a severely worn dentition: A dental technique.

J Prosthet Dent 2021;126:167-72.

42. **Perrin P, Eichenberger M, Neuhaus KW, Lussi A.**

Visual acuity and magnification devices in dentistry.

Swiss DentJ 2016;126(3):222 -35.

43. **Reuben HL, Apotheker H.**

Apical surgery with the dental microscope.

Oral Surg Oral Med Oral Pathol 1984;57:433-5.

44. **Robles M, Jurado CA, Azpiazu-Flores FX, Villalobos-Tinoco J,**

Afrashtehfar KI, Fischer NG.

An innovative 3D printed tooth reduction guide for precise dental ceramic veneers.

J Funct Biomater 2023;14(4):1 -9.

45. **Sadaqah NR.**

Ceramic laminate veneers: Materials advances and selection.

Open J Stomatol 2014;4:268-79.

46. **Salehi A.**

Ceramic veneers: A controllable preparation.

InfDent 2017;5:33-6.

47. **Sheets CG, Paquette JM, Hatate K.**

Masters of esthetic dentistry: The clinical microscope in an esthetic restorative practice.

J Esthet Restor Dent 2001;13:187-200.

48. **Silva BP, Stanley K, Gardee J.**

Laminate veneers: Preplanning and treatment using digital guided tooth preparation.

J Esthet Restor Dent 2020;32:150-60.

49. **Silva BP, Mahn Arteaga G, Mahn E.**

Predictable 3D guided adhesive bonding of porcelain veneers using 3D printed trays.

J Esthet Restor Dent 2021;33:692-701.

50. **Sitbon Y, Attathom T, St-Georges AJ.**

Minimal intervention dentistry II: Part 1. Contribution of the operating microscope to dentistry.

Br Dent J 2014;216:125-30.

51. **Soenen A, Pia JP, D'incau E.**

Conventional versus optical impressions.

Inf Dent 2015;29:2-7.

52. **Sola-Ruiz MF, Faus-Matoses I, Del Rio Highsmith J, Fons-Font A.**

Study of surface topography, roughness, and microleakage after dental preparation with different instrumentation.

Int J Prosthodont 2014;27:530-3.

53. **Yassmin F, Dent A.**

The use of digitally fabricated control guides in veneer preparation. A case study using Natural algorithms, Digital Smile Design (DSD) with CAD milled ceramics.

Aust Dent Pract 2020;10(2):148-53.

54. **Yu H, Zhao Y, Li J et al.**

Minimal invasive microscopic tooth preparation in esthetic restoration: A specialist consensus.

IntJ Oral Sci 2019;11:1-11.

55. **Yuzbasioglu E, Kurt H, Turunc R, Bilir H.**

Comparison of digital and conventional impression techniques: Evaluation of patients' perception, treatment comfort, effectiveness and clinical outcomes.

BMC Oral Health 2014;14:1-7.

56. **Zhang Y, Kelly JR.**

Dental ceramics for restoration and metal veneering.

Dent Clin North Am 2017;61:797-819.

Internet references

57. **Larousse dictionary.**

Definitions : Precision [Online].

[Accessed 22/12/2023], available from URL:

https://www.larousse.fr/dictionnaires/francais/pr% C3%A9cision/63354

58. **Digital MockUp**

SmileDesign [Online].

[Accessed 12/24/2023], available from URL :

https://www.mowbraydental.com.au/smile-design-digital-mockup.

59. **Dentistry Today.**

3D printed crown lengthening and reduction guide [Online].

[Accessed 10/01/2024], available from URL :

https://www.dentistrytoday.com/3d-printed-crown-lengthening-and-reduction-guide/

60. Le Fil Dentaire.

The operating microscope in endodontics [Online].

[Accessed 10/01/2024], available from URL :

https://www.lefildentaire.com/articles/clinique/endodontie/le-microscope-surgery-in-endodontics/

61. Newmed.

Dental microscope [Online].

[Accessed 15/01/2024], available from URL :

https://newmed.tn/fr/equipements/microscope-et-loupe/microscope-dental/microscope-dental-oms-2350.html

62. Medical Technologies .

ZEISS DPMI pico - Dental operating microscope [Online].

[Accessed 15/01/2024], available from URL :

https://www.zeiss.com/medi tec/en/products/microscopes-operatories/o pmi-pico.html.

63. Solowy MH.

Dental optical aids and binocular magnifiers [Online].

[Accessed on 25/01/2023], available from URL: https://www.eye-resolution.fr/3-dentaire.

(1) Cieslak, S. Veneers with and without dental preparation: current aspects.

(2) Bud, M.; Jitaru, S.; Lucaciu, O.; Korkut, B.; Dumitrascu-Timis, L.; Ionescu, C.; Cimpean, S.; Delean, A. The Advantages of the Dental Operative Microscope in Restorative Dentistry. *Med. Pharm. Rep.* **2020.** https://doi.org/10.15386/mpr-1662.

(3) van As, G. A. The Use of Extreme Magnification in Fixed Prosthodontics.

(4) Iman, R. Complications of ceramic veneers: a review of the literature over the past twenty years.

(5) Bud, M. G.; Pop, O. D.; Cîmpean, S. Benefits of Using Magnification in Dental Specialties - a Narrative Review. *Med. Pharm. Rep.* **2023,** *96* (3), 254-257. https://doi.org/10.15386/mpr-2556.

(6) *Definitions: precision - Dictionnaire defrançais Larousse.* https://www.larousse.fr/dictionnaires/francais/pr%C3%A9cision/63354 (accessed 2024-03-22).

(7) Pasceta, R. DOMENICO MASSIRONI, MD, DMD. . *and* **2004.**

(8) El-Mowafy, O.; El-Aawar, N.; El-Mowafy, N. Porcelain Veneers: An Update. *Dent. Med. Probl.* **2018,** *55* (2), 207-211. https://doi.org/10.17219/dmp/90729.

(9) Etienne, O.; Hajtô, J. Ceramic materials in "metal-free prosthetics"**. 2011,** No. 155.

(10) Sadaqah, N. R. Ceramic Laminate Veneers: Materials Advances and Selection. *OpenJ. Stomatol.* **2014,** *04* (05), 268-279. https://doi.org/10.4236/ojst.2014.45038.

(11) Gracis, S.; Thompson, V; Ferencz, J.; Silva, N.; Bonfante, E. A New Classification System for AllCeramic and Ceramic-like Restorative Materials. *Int. J. Prosthodont.* **2016,** *28* (3), 227-235. https://doi.org/10.11607/ijp.4244.

(12) Saint-Jean, S. J. Dental Glasses and Glass-Ceramics. In *Advanced Ceramicsfor Dentistry;* Elsevier, 2014; pp 255-277. https://doi.org/10.1016/B978-0-12-394619-5.00012-2.

(13) Ny, K.; Dm, P.; Ka, K. INTERESTS OF WAX UP IN THE DESIGN OF A COMPLEX FIXED PROTHETIC RESTORATION. **2017,***19.*

(14) Yu, H.;Zhao, Y.;Li, J.; Luo, T.; Gao, J.; Liu, H.;Liu, W.; Liu, F.;Zhao, K.; Liu, F.; Ma, C.; Setz, J. M.; Liang, S.; Fan, L.; Gao, S.; Zhu, Z.; Shen, J.; Wang, J.; Zhu, Z.; Zhou, X. Minimal Invasive MicroscopicTooth Preparation in Esthetic Restoration: A Specialist Consensus. *Int. J. OralSci.* **2019,***11* (3), 31. https://doi.org/10.1038/s41368-019-0057-y.

(15) AlSaleh, S.; Labban, M.; AlHariri, M.; Tashkandi, E. Evaluation of Self Shade Matching Ability of Dental Students Using Visual and Instrumental Means. *J. Dent.* **2012,** *40,* e82-e87. https://doi.Org/10.1016/j.jdent.2012.01.009.

(16) Derbabian, K.; Marzola, R.; Donovan, T. E.; Arcidiacono, A. The Science of Communicating the Art of Esthetic Dentistry. Part III: Precise Shade Communication. *J. Esthet. Restor. Dent.* **2001,***13* (3), 154-162. https://doi.Org/10.llll/j.1708-8240.2001.tb00258.x.

(17) Bergen, S. F.; McCasland, J. Dental Operatory Lighting and Tooth Color Discrimination. *J. Am. Dent.Assoc.* **1977,** 94(1), 130-134. https://doi.org/10.14219/jada.archive.1977.0264.

(18) Brewer, J. D.; Wee, A.; Seghi, R. Advances in Color Matching. *Dent. Clin. North Am.* **2004,** *48* (2), 341-358. https://doi.Org/10.1016/j.cden.2004.01.004.

(19) Paravina, R. D. Performance Assessment of Dental Shade Guides. *J. Dent.* **2009,** *37,* el5-e20. https://doi.Org/10.1016/j.jdent.2009.02.005.

(20) Corcodel, N.; Rammelsberg, P.; Jakstat, H.; Moldovan, O.; Schwarz, S.; Hassel, A. J. The Linear Shade Guide Design of Vita 3D-master Performs as Well as the Original Design of the Vita 3Dmaster. *J. OralRehabil.* **2010,** 37(11), 860-865. https://doi.org/10.1111/j,1365-2842.2010.02120.x.

(21) Haddad, H. J.; Jakstat, H. A.; Arnetzl, G.; Borbely, J.; Vichi, A.; Dumfahrt, H.; Renault, P.;Corcodel, N.; Pohlen, B.; Marada, G.; De Parga, J. A. M. V.; Reshad, M.; Klinke, T. U.; Hannak, W. B.; Paravina, R. D. Does Gender and Experience Influence Shade Matching Quality?!. *Dent.* **2009,** *37,* e40-e44. https://doi.Org/10.1016/j.jdent.2009.05.012.

(22) Salehi, A. The ceramic veneer: a controllable preparation. **2017.**

(23) Magne, P.; Belser, U. C. Novel Porcelain Laminate Preparation Approach Driven by a Diagnostic Mock-Up. 7. *Esthet. Restor. Dent.* **2004,***16* (1), 7-16. https://doi.org/10.1111/j,1708- 8240.2004.tb00444.x.

(24) Alexandre, D. K. K. KOUAME K A, KONE T, PESSON D M, DIDIA E L, KONATE N Y, DJEREDOU K B. **2014,** *21.*

(25) Hosmalin, R. Design and production of fixed prostheses using indirect CAD/CAM.

(26) Soenen, A.; Pia, J.-P. Conventional impressions versus optical impressions. **2015.**

(27) Hamalian, T. A.; Nasr, E.; Chidiac, J. J. Impression Materials in Fixed Prosthodontics: Influence of Choice on Clinical Procedure: Impression Materials: A Review. *J. Prosthodont.* **2011,** *20* (2), 153160. https://doi.Org/10.llll/j.1532-849X.2010.00673.x.

(28) Hamlett, K. The Art of Veneer Cementation. *Alpha Omegan* **2009,***102* (4), 128-132. https://doi.Org/10.1016/j.aodf.2009.10.008.

(29) ALGhazali, N.; Laukner, J.; Burnside, G.; Jarad, F. D.; Smith, P. W.; Preston, A. J. An Investigation into the Effect of Try-in Pastes, Uncured and Cured Resin Cements on the Overall Color of Ceramic Veneer Restorations: An in Vitro Study. *J. Dent.* **2010,** *38,* e78-e86. https://doi.Org/10.1016/j.jdent.2010.08.013.

(30) Marques, S.; Ribeiro, P.; Gama, C.; Herrero-Climent, M. Digital Guided Veneer Preparation: A Dental Technique. 7. *Prosthet. Dent. 2022,* S002239132200381X. https://doi.Org/10.1016/j.prosdent.2022.04.035.

(31) *Smile Design /Digital MockUp.* Mowbray Dental, https://www.mowbraydental.com.au/smile-design-digital-mockup (accessed 2024-03-22).

(32) Caponi, L.; Raslan, F.; Roig, M. Fabrication of a Facially Generated Tooth Reduction Guide for

Minimally Invasive Preparations: A Dental Technique. *J. Prosthet. Dent. 2022,127* (5), 689-694. https://doi.Org/10.1016/j.prosdent.2020.ll.030.

(33) *3D Printed Crown Lengthening and Reduction Guide - Dentistry Today.* https://www.dentistrytoday.com/3d-pnnted-crown-lengthening-and-reduction-guide/ (accessed 2024-03-22).

(34) Yassmin, F.; Dent, A. The Use of Digitally Fabricated Control Guides in Veneer Preparation. A Case Study Using Natural Algorithms, Digital Smile Design (DSD) with CAD Milled Ceramics. **2020.**

(35) Robles, M.; Jurado, C. A.; Azpiazu-Flores, F. X.; Villalobos-Tinoco, J.; Afrashtehfar, K. I.; Fischer, N. G. An Innovative 3D Printed Tooth Reduction Guide for Precise Dental Ceramic Veneers. *J. Fund. Biomater.* **2023,***14* (4), 216. https://doi.org/10.3390/jftl4040216.

(36) Yuzbasioglu, E.; Kurt, H.; Turunc, R.; Bilir, H. Comparison of Digital and Conventional Impression Techniques: Evaluation of Patients' Perception, Treatment Comfort, Effectiveness and Clinical Outcomes. *BMC OralHealth* **2014,***14* (1), 10. https://doi.org/10.1186/1472-6831-14-10.

(37) Silva, B. P. D.; Stanley, K.; Gardee, J. Laminate Veneers: Preplanning and Treatment Using Digital Guided Tooth Preparation. *J. Esthet. Restor. Dent.* **2020,** *32* (2), 150-160. https://doi.org/10.llll/jerd.12571.

(38) Carvalho, T. F.; Lima, J. F. M.; de-Matos, J. D. M.; Lopes, G. D. R. S.; Vasconcelos, J. E. L. D.; Zogheib, L. V.; de-Castro, D. S. M. Evaluation of the Accuracy of Conventional and Digital Methods OfObtaining Dental Impressions. *Int. J. Odontostomatol.* **2018,***12* (4), 368-375. https://doi.org/10.4067/S0718-381X2018000400368.

(39) Cazier, S.; Moussally, C. Description of the various digital impression systems. **2013.**

(40) Duret, F.; Pélissier, B. Different impression methods in dental CAD/CAM.

(41) Christensen, G. J. Will Digital Impressions Eliminate the Current Problems With Conventional Impressions? 7 *Am. Dent. Assoc.* **2008,***139* (6), 761-763. https://doi.org/10.14219/jada.archive.2008.0258.

(42) Cicciù, M.; Fiorillo, L.; D'Amico, C.; Gambino, D.; Amantia, E. M.; Laino, L.; Crimi, S.; Campagna, P.; Bianchi, A.; Herford, A. S.; Cervino, G. 3D Digital Impression Systems Compared with Traditional Techniques in Dentistry: A Recent Data Systematic Review. **2020.**

(43) Ng, J.; Ruse, D.; Wyatt, C. A Comparison of the Marginal Fit of Crowns Fabricated with Digital and Conventional Methods. 7. *Prosthet. Dent.* **2014,***112* (3), 555-560. https://doi.Org/10.1016/j.prosdent.2013.12.002.

(44) Hampé-Kautz, V.; Salehi, A.; Senger, B.; Etienne, O. A Comparative in Vivo Study of New Shade Matching Procedures. *Int. J. Comput. Dent.* **2020,** *23* (4), 317-323.

(45) Liberato, W. F.; Barreto, I. C.; Costa, P. P.; De Almeida, C. C.; Pimentel, W; Tiossi, R. A Comparison between Visual, Intraoral Scanner, and Spectrophotometer Shade Matching: A Clinical Study. 7. *Prosthet. Dent.* **2019,***121* (2), 271-275.

https://doi.Org/10.1016/j.prosdent.2018.05.004.

(46) Mohammed, A. O.; Mohammed, G. S.; Mathew, M.; Alzarea, B.; Bandela, V. Shade Selection in Esthetic Dentistry: A Review. *Cureus* **2022.** https://doi.org/10.7759/cureus.23331.

(47) Chu, S. J.; Trushkowsky, R. D.; Paravina, R. D. Dental Color Matching Instruments and Systems. Review of Clinical and Research Aspects. *J. Dent.* **2010,** *38,* e2-el6. https://doi.Org/10.1016/j.jdent.2010.07.001.

(48) Corcodel, N.; Helling, S.; Rammelsberg, P.; Hassel, A. J. Metameric Effect between Natural Teeth and the Shade Tabs of a Shade Guide. *Eur. J. OralSci.* **2010,***118* (3), 311-316. https://doi.Org/10.llll/j.1600-0722.2010.00730.x.

(49) Silva, B. P.; Mahn Arteaga, G.; Mahn, E. Predictable 3D Guided Adhesive Bonding of Porcelain Veneers Using 3D Printed Trays. *J. Esthet. Restar. Dent.* **2021,** *33* (5), 692-701. https://doi.org/10.llll/jerd.12795.

(50) Sitbon, Y; Attathom, T.; St-Georges, A. J. Minimal Intervenhon Denhstry II: Part 1. Contribuhon ofthe Operahng Microscope to Denhstry. *Br. Dent. J.* **2014,** *216* (3), 125-130. https://doi.org/10.1038/sj.bdj.2014.48.

(51) Burkhardt, R. Orientahons nouvelles en chirurgie plastique parodontale. *109.*

(52) Low, J. F.; Dom, T. N. M.; Baharin, S. A. Magnihcahon in Endodonhcs: A Review of Its Applicahon and Acceptance among Dental Prachhoners. *Eur. J. Dent.* **2018,***12* (04), 610-616. https://doi.org/10.4103/ejd.ejd_248_18.

(53) Forgie, A. H. Magnihcahon: What Is Available, and Will It Aid Your Clinical Prachce? *Dent. Update* **2001,** *28* (3), 125-130. https://doi.Org/10.12968/denu.2001.28.3.125.

(54) *The operating microscope in endodontics.* https://www.lefildentaire.com/articles/clinique/endodonhe/le-microscope-operatoire-en-endodonhe/ (accessed 2024-03-22).

(55) Aboalshamat, K.; Daoud, O.; Mahmoud, L. A.; Attal, S.; Alshehri, R.; Bin Othman, D.; Alzahrani, R. Prachces and Affitudes of Dental Loupes and Their Relahonship to Musculoskeletal Disorders among Dental Prachhoners. *Int. J. Dent.* **2020,** *2020,* 1-7. https://doi.org/10.1155/2020/8828709.

(56) Reuben, H. L.; Apotheker, H. Apical Surgery with the Dental Microscope. *OralSurg. Oral Med. OralPathol.* **1984,** 57(4), 433-435. https://doi.org/10.1016/0030-4220(84)90164-6.

(57) Carr, G. B. Microscopes in Endodonhcs. *J. Calif. Dent. Assoc.* **1992,** *20* (11), 55-61.

(58) Massironi, D.; Romeo, G.; Pascetta, R.; Bywaters, L. C.; Goates, B. *Precision in Dental Esthetics: Clinical andLaboratory Procedures;* Quintessenza Edizioni, 2007.

(59) Cordero, I. Understanding and maintaining an operating microscope.

(60) Mamoun, J.; Wilkinson, M. E.; Feinbloom, R. Technical Aspects and Clinical Usage of Keplerian and Galilean Binocular Surgical Loupe Telescopes Used in Denhstry or Medicine.

(61) *(https://newmed.tn/fr/equipements/microscope-et-loupe/microscope-dentaire/microscope-dental-oms-2350.html) - Google search.* https://www.google.com/search?sca_esv=68ac34d273474b3b&sxsrf=ACQVn09IBI617AINKI J4EA _8IFZNei0PzA:1711135343004&q=(https://newmed.tn/fr/equipements/microscope-et- loupe/microscope-dental/microscope-dental-oms-

2350.html)&tbm=isch&source=lnms&sa=X&ved=2ahUKEwjhlKDyy4iFAxVygP0HHZy7BlUQ0 pQJ egQIDhAB&biw=1366&bih=641&dpr=l#imgrc=rR8_Ve-NiKn0bM (accessed 2024-03-22).

(62) *ZEISS OPMI pico - Dental operating microscope.* https://www.zeiss.com/meditec/fr/produits/microscopes-operatoires/opmi-pico.html (accessed 2024-03-22).

(63) Sheets, C. G.; Paquette, J. M.; Hatate, K. Masters of Esthehc Denhstry: THE CLINICAL MICROSCOPE IN AN ESTHETIC RESTORATIVE PRACTICE. *J. Esthet. Restor. Dent.* **2001,** *13* (3), 187200. https://doi.Org/10.llll/j.1708-8240.2001.tb00262.x.

(64) Pascotto, R. C.; Beneffi, A. R. The Clinical Microscope and Direct Composite Veneer. *Oper. Dent.* **2010,** *35* (2), 246-249. https://doi.org/10.2341/09-118-T.

(65) James, T.; Gilmour, A. S. Magnifying Loupes in Modern Dental Prachce: An Update. *Dent. Update* **2010,** 37(9), 633-636. https://doi.Org/10.12968/denu.2010.37.9.633.

(66) Juggins, K. J. Current Products and Prachce: The BiggerThe Better: Can Magnihcahon Aid Orthodonhc Clinical Prachce?!. *Orthod.* **2006,** *33* (1), 62-66. https://doi.org/10.1179/146531205225021420.

(67) Perrin, P.; Eichenberger, M. 222 RESEARCH AND SCIENCE. **2016,** *126.*

(68) *Dental optical aids and binocular loupes - Eye Resolution,* https://www.eye- resoluhon.fr/3-dentaire (accessed 2024-03-22).

(69) Brunton, P. A.; Aminian, A.; Wilson, N. H. F. Tooth Preparahon Technlques for Porcelain Laminate Veneers. *Restorative Dent.* **2000,** *189* (5).

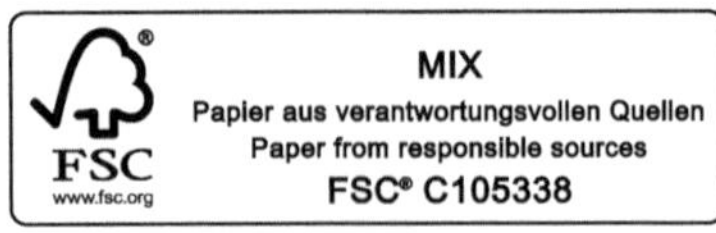

Printed by Books on Demand GmbH, Norderstedt / Germany